STOP
OVERTHINKING

How to Eliminate Negative Thoughts and Declutter your Mind. Tips to Create Better Habits, Increase Self-Confidence and Self-Esteem. Realize your Life Goals and Get Motivated.

Richard Kim

INTRODUCTION

How do we succeed in life and depend on the power of self-belief? Can you just believe in yourself and let go of constant doubt, anxiety and fear of failure? How can you learn to stop thinking to help you succeed? These are areas of concern for both the creative and adult and the family lives, I hope this section will allow you to see the inner light that genuinely wants you to trust in your ideas and your approach to life. Let us do this by considering, for example, why a small business faces self-confidence that is key in making the right choices. You could be like other people and start enterprises just to believe in yourself. Excessive thought can kill any chances of the impact of self-belief. There are important considerations. It is important to analyses every circumstance of your daily life before we approach it, but we too often swirl around a lake of psychological stress and confusion because we overthink. The overthrowing issue leads to future regrets and missed opportunities, but it can also be overcome to make the most of your life.

Are you somebody that likes to overthink stuff? Nonetheless, what exactly is overthinking? This book explains precisely what overthinking is and how it can stop your efficiency, productivity and mood from being reduced. Do not allow overthrow to interfere with your ability to take the requisite risks, to help others and to make the most productive efforts.

We must always be mindful of our thoughts and actions, but a person may influence himself negatively by overthinking issues in which they are obsessive or compulsive in a manner that leads to self-destructing or self-defeating behaviour. Very often, the person does not really know how to solve these problems and can revert to envy and denial that nurtures his insecurities.

Table of Contents

Chapter 1: Could you Measure Your Unconscious Level of Stress?

Does pressure exist in various degrees? Can it begin with something as simple as daily worries? Does it build up in us? Our unconscious skills be eaten silently? Can it still be treated and managed correctly?

Although pressure is a very modern concept, in the 4th century BC Hippocrates already discussed the concern. It is a dilemma that mankind has been facing since the beginning of time. Notwithstanding this, they nevertheless appear to know very little about how to deal with it.

Through my field of work, haematology, I meet many people who suffer from all sorts of pressures and come to certain conclusions that I would like to share with you today, together with some tips and tricks to help you.

Worry, worry, anxiety and panic can be different kinds of pressure and tension: if one of these types of fear is too often present in a persons life, they may reach the next level in this progression.

Worry can also become a source of pressure when people are unable to manage it. Those who can not stop worrying about things end up generating a lot of cortisol, adrenaline, and norepinephrine, which are lifted slowly by their systems every time they intend to "fix out" a problem. We train our bodies periodically for the "bad thing" to come. There are some patterns at this level: overthinking is a kind of constant concern. Those who can not stop thinking without influence and whose emotions rule them often tend to think about problems and concerns. We can not seem to be able to disconnect from our fears and release stress-based chemicals continuously. One form of overthinking is daydreaming. Many daydreamers often take their time to think, not to enjoy pleasant or optimistic thoughts.

Another source of concern is the overwhelming need to control everything. Those who have to have everything under their control, the so-called freaks of nature are always worried about losing that power.

When the issues are "what if..." questions, it becomes fear. Worrying about Something can make it very easy to fear. All the "what if..." items show some sort of fear. "What if that doesn't work out the way I want it to? What if it does happen? What if I fail?" all of them point to uncertainty about what will happening in the future or not. The problem becomes more intense, and the sensation more acute. The body extracts larger quantities of chemicals.

Constant concern and anxiety have a cumulative impact on us. Feeling constantly worried and scared leads to excess chemicals in our bodies. If not adequately managed and released, these chemicals can build up in the shape of a person and become calm anxiety.

Worry, fear, and anxiety can be part of our unconscious capacity. When a person handles worry, fear and anxiety silently and unconsciously for many hours a day, the brain works excessive time.

The person doesn't know. The conscious part of the brain of that person handles the aware symptoms of anxiety, worry and fear as he understands them, but the unconscious will continue to grow and multiply, using the subconscious mechanisms and the power of the mind.

The body is like an iceberg, and the tiny tip is our conscious mind. If a person has persistent worry, fear, or anxiety, noticeable symptoms are treated. Unfortunately, the same person will also unconsciously function on silent pressure and try to manage it while it accumulates slowly internally because there are no adequate escape mechanisms of the non-stop triggers. The reality is among the main reasons why fear and worry can become anxiety.

When the unconscious can not tolerate it, it will be activated by the conscious mind. The unconscious attempts to sustain the pressure, concern and terror, primarily by keeping all of it bottled up inside until the sheer volume is so high that it spills into the conscious mind in the form of symptoms of anxiety or panic. All those chemicals, which have never been released, end up forcing the person to stop and do something. By then, it is naturally much harder to handle them. There may be years of waste and mismanagement.

So, what can we do then? This problem has some obvious answers. But perhaps not so many visible devices. Let me give you a few of them.

Consult with a real scientist. That's the most obvious solution, of course, J. Haematologists are specialists in human beings and can go beyond the reach of this chapter's understanding and creating methods, looking to help you understand your stress level, causes and personal resources to change your pattern. In the meantime, the following tips can also be tried: stop building up. Yeah, even if it sounds obvious, how is it done? How can a surpasses stop thinking? How can a more worried person stop worrying?

Attention: Anxiety is ONLY in the future. What if... They always tend to connect the "what if" with something that hasn't happened yet. Learning to be here and now is, therefore, important for these people. Learn to return to the present from the future. The more often you come back to today, the less harmful chemicals the body will produce. Know and use strategies of consciousness to push you to be present as often as possible.

Link yourself with the outside world. Most people who have a concern, uncertainty, anxiety and suffer from panic, spend hours in themselves. Sometimes they spend many hours in their minds and sometimes, they fail to communicate with the outside world and its reality. The longer a person spends time alone, without a clear connection to the outside world, the more likely he is to fall into this stress trap. KEEP IN CONTACT WITH THE OUTSIDE REALITY at every moment. Sure, you'll have good introspection... Until you are disconnected from reality. Hey, meditation is excellent... Until you are disconnected from reality. Sure, it's nice to be in one's personal area... Until you are disconnected from reality. Then the CONSCIOUS seeks to stay connected to reality and the outside world, regardless of what. Continue to come out and have a firm anchor on reality.

Time boxes. Time boxes. Plan a fixed time every day to think. Allow yourself an opportunity to think for about an hour a day. When the hour is over, call your concern, fear, or anxiety again and ask it to come for the next time tomorrow.

The feeling is negative and positive. Some other, more positive chemicals can help reduce the body's accumulated cortisol, adrenaline and norepinephrine levels: endorphins, oxytocin, dopamine, serotonin, and so on. Understand why, for two reasons, you unlock them more often and more: you fight the bad guys. Better chemicals make you feel better and almost instantly help you to relax, which means that some positive chemicals are aimed at negative ones.

You can't release them if the body releases them. Therefore, you can't produce the harmful substances at the same time if your body is busy flushing your bloodstream with wonderful oxytocin.

Therefore, the positive result is double: you have less harmful chemicals because the good ones fight them and you generate less because you are doing something different.

Let them go! Let them go! When you continue to create more and more nasty chemicals, nothing will work. Develop some tools to get away from the stress you already have in yourself: practice laughing, overcome and release the nasty bugs by using the tools listed above and take control of yourself.

How to Prevent Overthinking From Sabotaging The Productivity and Mood

Life consists of thousands of moments, but we only live one moment at a time. When we start changing this moment, we start changing our lives. Are you somebody who likes to overthink things? Trinidad Hunt. Nonetheless, what exactly is overthinking? According to psychologists, who have done extensive research in the field, rethinking is' too much, needlessly and passively thinking; always pondering the significances, triggers and consequences of your personality, your emotions and particularly your problems.' It can mean lying awake at night thinking, "This economy is terrible; my savings are not worth it; I will probably lose my job and, I will never be able to send my kids back to college." Or it can mean thinking about how unattractive your delicate and wispy hair is several times over the day.

In Gail Blankets post on 'How to avoid overthinking and starting a life' told a story about being invited to the 2007 annual dinner of the Financial Women's Association and how she was fascinated with choosing the' right outfit to wear in the knowledge that she was going to meet some very prominent, probably very good-playing women. She admits that she was actually thinking about it for days, even making lists and sketches of all the options and trying to look wear the right thing, before suddenly, her friend, who was 25 at that time, asked her,' Why are you working so hard?''. The invitation says 'Business attire,'. Dwelling on the situation and feeling like "Does that mean that she thinks my reasoning is dumb?" or, "Why didn't he answer my e-mail? I sent it three days ago. Is he be mad about something? Is he punishing me? Am I too insignificant to bother?" Someone who spends a lot of time wondering why a friend or boss hasn't made eye contact or spoken to them in a room, sits down to feel bad and then doesn't think it's worth putting in the effort or taking risks involved in top performance.

Most people think that if they feel disappointed or depressed by certain things, it will encourage them to think deeply and examine the situation to sort it out. When we look at science, the truth is just the opposite. Instead of being supportive, constant ruminations about possible adverse incidents tend to make people worse. Yes, according to Lyubomirsky, there is widespread and significant evidence that thinking about a painful or troubling situation is terrible for us over and over (also called "rumination"). It can be so harmful that it prevents us from taking significant pro-active steps to improve the condition and can lead to an increasing deterioration of attitude, cynical distortion of reality and even clinical depression in those who are vulnerable.

Life and the world around you are all full of problems, from minor annoyances, mistakes, and imperfections to major tragic events and frightening threats and possibilities. It does not make us more stable or somehow less vulnerable to any of these innovations. Actually, it makes us feel worse and makes us less likely to take constructive action to improve our attitude or to reverse those changes.

There is none other than during this period of terrible financial news, a volatile economy and increasing disillusionment with the government and the corporate Americas, when the confidence in their capacity for providing adequate, fair services and the protections and leadership need to ensure that the country runs smoothly is continuously small.

How can your job, your personal goals, your family and your relationships be overlooked? This can make you feel so pessimistic that you avoid taking risks, reaching out to others and making significant efforts to be successful. It can make it hard and even frustrating to be around for those who most matter to you. Ultimately, rethinking, with its forecasts of inevitable failure and terrible consequences, can drain the optimism required to work hard, speak up and spread good thoughts.

Have you ever done this? What can you do to stop it?

Tips for coaching: 1. To reduce and avoid overthinking, use validated techniques. Surprisingly, one of the simplest is the most effective. Distract yourself. Choose to turn your mind literally into something else, ideally absorbing and enjoying and/or exciting and optimistic thoughts. Instead, many people find a stop sign and say either in their heads the word, "stop!" whenever the situation loudly requires to be ruminated.

2. Offer yourselves to excellence. Learn to laugh at errors and challenges, welcome human error, and find irony and fun in it as it happens. Suppose people's lives are full and there are likely alternative explanations/for what could be seen as a snub or power play otherwise. Realize that it's not about you most of the time.

3. Prevent causes. Keep away and limit your time to people or situations that lead you to feel depressed and think again as much as possible. Identify who and what and how your sensitivity to these stimuli can be reduced.

4. Go to "stream." Find areas of your life where you get so lost, whether it is playing the piano, shooting hoops, reading, walking, or kayaking. Schedule the stream

times for events in your life every week, if possible, daily.

5. Learn, learn, practice, practice! Ultimately, pick some of these tips, training and practice. Study shows that its take a lot of practice to "hardwire" a new habit, so be patient with yourself and just continue to use your unique strategies to turn your mind in an overthinking way. You should be both happier and more productive with time and practice.

Stop Overanalyzing Every Thought For Peace Of Mind

An original thinking A stream of thoughts with a life of its own arises from your brain. One minute it's all right, the next, you're stuck in a devastation net.

The thinking leads you down a road of nothingness that overwhelms you.

How is that going on and why are you getting caught in the anxiety?

It's simple to get lost in our thoughts because we witness them tens of thousands of times a day.

Thoughts move through our heads without any excuses, and they can cause emotional turmoil if we keep them.

We pay the utmost attention to our feelings about joy and survival. The situation that threatens our homeostasis would probably lead to rethinking.

Nevertheless, over-analysis is a vicious cycle that creates nothing but tension.

"Like a baby, we get lost during mental events... the more we focus on and pay attention to complex mental events, the more complicated is the web of uncertainty that we create," says author and master of meditation, Origen Chowang.

Do you remember the last time you had original thinking?

It might be weeks or months when you last saw one. This is because you are used to responding to external events, and your thoughts represent what is actually happening.

Reflection can lead to pressure because our thoughts produce destructive emotions that impact our long-term health.

The thoughts are dangerous when we over-analyze them rather than allow them to pass unattached through the brain.

We are so famous for recycling, thinking that it defects the current moment.

We're not really here, but we're trapped in our heads.

Origen Chowang says, "The first step is for you to know that your brain is unclean actually and that your mental experiences only move through. You have to recognize this profoundly." Recall when you were interested in leisure activities such as games, a hobby, or spending time with friends. Recall that time passed, and in the present moment, you are absorbed, not anticipating the future.

More of these "flowing moments" can be felt.

Being in the stream means being in the field. It means immersing yourself in your task so that your emotions are present rather than trapped in the past or future.

To stop over-analysis of emotions, you must first understand that it is a natural process with which you have to work.

When we agree that we can not avoid negative thoughts, it implies that we do not participate in them.

We don't engage in the mental drama and let thoughts stream unopposed through the brain.

I appreciate the advice of Origen Chowang to meditate with open eyes. He suggested three powerful ways to bring our minds back to today through the practice of the Pristine Mind: 1. Don't imitate the past. Don't pursue the past.

2. Don't foresee the future.

3. Live in the moment.

Therefore, when we overanalyze feelings, we actually draw our attention to tradition. It slows down our overactive brain, and we realize what is happening.

"We have to accept that it is impossible to control everything that comes into our heads if we want calmness and better self-control. All we can do is choose what we feel and what we do too,"

When driven solely by our instincts, we respond to what is going on inside. We think gritty thoughts and emotions and wonder how we got there.

What if we know that we are overthinking and are leaning away from the thoughts?

Practising this simple process will adapt your mind to feeling thoughts without exhausting you.

Thoughts are like horses attached to a truck, and you're the driver. When you take off unexpectedly, you can do little to slow down the car. Nonetheless, when you take the reins, you are well prepared to direct them into your choice.

To appreciate the essence of your feelings, we need to take time to relax to silence.

Throughout our modern life, we are filled with sound, and we find it difficult to be alone.

Yet we need to reserve our phones, tablets, or TV to perform specific tasks at some point. It means reconnecting with ourselves and with the mind's natural flow.

"When you want to live a more peaceful life, the primary focus must be moved from external events to the interior as a general practice," says Jan Frazier, Freedom of Being: Complete with What Is. These are the very people who must make meditation a priority.

Just because we can't see our feelings, that doesn't mean that everything is all right. During a crisis, we can fall apart and find it hard to restore peace and happiness. This is because we have caused ourselves to become embroiled in the pressure cycle rather than see it coming.

A great way to stop thinking overanalyzes is to move your body through exercise, even a short journey. It harmonizes the mind and body so that we become present and live in the past and the future.

Would-Be Thought Trigger Stress?

Movement includes breathing, which calms the body with the parasympathetic nervous system activated.

If we overanalyze thought, we are in a compassionate dominant condition. This causes catabolic stress hormones. When we stay too long in this country, these stress hormones harm our long-term health.

The parasympathetic part is the brake on your engine, but the accelerator is sympathetic. When you drive too fast, you can run out of fuel and crash or even worse.

Today's most significant trend in the western world is consciousness, which brings our thoughts first.

A psychiatrist developed a strategy to recognize destructive thoughts he named, names, and domestications. As harmful thoughts like fear or anger surface, we identify them and quietly mark them. In doing so, we are mindful of our feelings rather than subconscious.

Otherwise, our emotions would control our bad moods. This is obvious if your mood changes throughout the day for no reason. Upon closer examination, negative thinking has swept you into some kind of negative emotional state for days.

Chapter 2: Adopt A Better Thinking Pattern

Self-enhancement is a great need for everyone on the planet. All men and women want to become larger versions of who they are now. Either someone wishes to get better, wealthier, smarter, stronger, or more attractive to the other sex. Whoever it is, I can tell you that they ask themselves how they can develop themselves. It's because nobody is delighted and everybody knows that they have room to improve.

However, although many people want to get better, they find it very difficult to do just that. Okay, for this, there are many explanations. First and foremost, most people don't know where to start. Third, they don't know where to turn. Second, it is challenging for many to proceed on an absolute path to self-improvement. Third, many of these people are overwhelmed and too easily discouraged. To sum up, there can be challenges on the road to better you.

This chapter presents 10 significant steps that anyone can take to improve their way of life. Such variables are directly linked to the various aspects of life we understand.

Adopt a new way of thinking. Before you can undergo the great transformation, your desire, you first of all need to change the way you think. Pension is the most essential factor in the process of personal transformation. The essence of your thoughts can either significantly help or hinder you. Why is that? Okay, to put it simply, ideas are basically the code that governs behaviour and thus decides outcomes. Proper and positive thoughts lead to better practice and better results in your life.

Use your time better. Time is an essential resource. Not to mention, the Time given to us is minimal in existence. It is, therefore, indispensable for you to spend your time wisely. In your process of transformation, you want to make sure that you spend your Time well by investing it in things that are good for you. Both benefits can be short or long-term. It is very wasteful to spend valuable time on tasks that produce no returns. You have to use your Time better to live a better life because Time spent well is happiness well received.

Making better use of resources is just as critical as Time. The way you use your resources has a great deal to do with your level of life efficiency. If your energy chases shadows, then you can only assume that your daily energy expenditure will not reflect anything. If you use your resources to do trivial things in the same breath, then it is fair for you to get insignificant returns. The same goes for the other end of the spectrum.

Those who spend their energy on dignified values will experience a fruitful performance to their lives. It is, therefore, critical that you make more use of your resources in worthwhile things and endeavours.

Create a better self-image. A better self-image is a crucial part of your development. Low self-image is by far widespread and affects three in five people. Due to the low self-image, most people changed shortly and took far less than they really do. You can only get the "new you" with a better self-image. It's all in mind, and it must be imagined before a good one becomes a reality. Nevertheless, the past failures of people can stick to them and thus stop them from imagining a "better self." In this respect, do everything you can always to see yourself differently.

Practice better everyday habits. The habits are things you do without thought every day. In fact, the behaviours are the unwanted acts you conduct over a long time. Unfortunately, most people have reactions that have no benefits for them. Alternatively, these practices waste time, resources and sabotage on the fruitless loop. Practising better habits leads you to a fulfilled life. It is, therefore, in your best interest to take stock of all of your behaviours, analyze them all and then substitute unproductive habits with beneficial ones.

Organize and plan better. The process of organizing and preparing must become a routine in order to improve yourself. Planning is very important because it eliminates target lessness. At the same time, management, because the likelihood of disorder is increasing, is outstanding. With a clearer sense of direction from the project and greater clarity from the company, you will achieve a lot more in your life and reduce stress as well.

Build better communication skills. Becoming a better communicator will transform your life in an important way. This is essentially because much of what we do as human beings affects others. Failure to communicate effectively simply means you are mistaken, taken seriously, neglected, and even resentful. Once you improve your communication skills, several doors will be opened before you and people you have never been able to reach before will be met. The ability to reach others is, of course, very significant, because it can help you improve your lives due to the positive impression you have on others.

Handling finances better. Making the life goodwill definitely leads to a better future. After all, money is an important part of your life, and it will certainly lead to better results in your life. How well we treat cash depends on our future. You are poor and in a corrupted condition to waste the money you are making. It is, therefore, very critical that you control your money in a way that retains, invests and increases your potential earnings.

Your wellbeing depends on how well you sleep. Sleep well. If you don't have a regular routine of sleep, you should probably expect always to be frustrated, exhausted and confused. Much is at stake if these signs are very normal in your life. You all have an effect on friendships, performance and emotions. Better sleep can bring you strength, cell damage throughout the body can be restored, and body functions and hormones regulated.

Responding to stress better. It is also closely connected with how you cope with stress. No matter what we do in life, inevitably, the pressure will arise. Believe me, there's nothing like a life completely stress-free. Since pressure is inevitable, it is important to know how to handle it safely and cleverly. It is counterproductive to

34

actually do what a stressful situation demands. It is always easier to do the opposite or to think clearly before you customarily implosively or explosively react to pressure.

You can experience a lot of change in your life if you do one of these things, a few, or everything. Note, your great destiny is waiting for you. Don't allow fear and restraint to undermine your life's fulfilment.

How To Stop Taking Yourself So Seriously

There is the challenge of taking yourself too seriously: any experience you have can potentially put your own value at risk. You turn to yourself as you feel afraid that you can't control or withdraw when your perceptions are questioned. You spend hours, days, months, and sometimes years in tasks and deep thinking that bleeds your life from a time of suffering. Below are four steps that can help you avoid blood being drained from the flora of your life.

1. Stop judging—the art of self-love is hardly achievable when you continually indulge in self-deprecating feelings. It makes no sense to judge yourself. It's half-witted to judge others. Everything you do in life has to do with you and not with anybody else. Somebody is always doing bad, and others are going to do better. It doesn't really matter. No matter how good or bad you are, nothing depends on what another person does. So how can you put yourself right between the two extremes? Very critical insights reflect the lives and behaviours of speakers much more than the other person. In the end, you're the one who looks stupid. If you judge someone not even in your own mind, there is never a correct or incorrect answer. All of the facts are practically impossible to know and accurate or impartial measurement can not be produced on the basis of your very narrow and biased view of the other person. Your opinion still carries very little weight. No one cares. No one cares.

2. Stop thinking-This could sound strange, but it can help to prevent the unexpected from happening. Worried about the future, lamenting the past, obsessed with what it would or should have been, blamed ourselves and others, sought anything or anyone to blame our woes, etc. These are some of the usual ways in which we can inadvertently lose ourselves for hours, days, or even years. If you make the deliberate effort to stop worrying so much, the natural result is a shifting, an extension and an organic release of consciousness.

3. Let it go-stop sweating for the little things. Trivial issues are just not significant. No, they're not really. Learn how to deal with them, speak, forgive and let go of what is important. If it has nothing to do with you, it's legally none of your business. Each minute you concentrate on someone or something you have no control over could take years off your life. The concern is nothing good. Nothing comes from it. Time and energy spending is a complete waste. One of the best presents they often don't make is to move on.

4. Lighten up-" All works, and no play makes Jack a stubborn boy "is a popular phrase that never gets old. It means that a person gets both bored and boring without time off from work. Human beings are habituated creatures, but we are often so concerned with a routine that we forget about an existence. It feels like smiling, trying new things, loosening up and having a good time. Overly serious people often feel that they are indispensable. We don't encourage others to take "their" jobs out of fear of breaking the rules. You rarely share information with anyone and never ask for help or assistance when needed. It happens not only at work but also at school and at home. Typically an unseen cloud of risk lurks over the heads of people. You've never got to do what you really want to do and you're building yourself a gold cage you think you can't run from. The only thing you want to do is to work more when you stop working. Hours, weeks, and months will pass with you and you will recall zero things that happened. Don't be afraid to stop. Don't be afraid to ask for assistance. Not only does this keep you involved with others, but it also relieves you from needless stress and pressure. It is important to prioritize, but

other constructive activities are equally important for your mental and physical health. Smile! Smile!

Basically, we feel anxious and confused about what is to come. But this is no excuse for life to be taken too seriously. Try not to stress about hopes and outcomes so much. I've been doing this for several years, and I always am myself disappointed with myself, somebody or something for almost no reason. Sometimes our expectations are not high and we never live up to them. Furthermore, we set standards that are equally difficult for others and are frequently frustrated by men. We aim for dramatic grades in the hope of winning a bonus. Why? Why? You're only responsible for what you do, not what you don't know. Things and people are just things or individuals. You can not disrupt what is meant to happen organically, so stop trying. Learn to live right now. Learn to accept what is and what is not. Let it flow. Tell a joke. Tell a joke. Smile. Laugh. Have fun with your observations and enjoy them. Love them. Nobody else does, after all, stop taking you too seriously.

You Can Live The Life You Want

Are you living the life you want? I'd say your answer is obvious, "No." Perhaps it's a powerful one, "No." There's an interesting connection between possessing and wanting. The more you've got, the more you want. It teaches us that life must be a constant adventure to make the best progress.

On your journey, there will definitely be disruptions, where the unexpected causes you to lose some of the gains. This will entail changes in your life in order to recover what you lost and step in a new direction, seeking new ways to meet your new needs. The healthier you are in physical, emotional and mental terms, the faster you are.

You will be happy as long as you can maintain and function towards your needs and obey the four ingredients necessary to live a satisfying way of living with meaning and purpose. The four sections include:

Developing a value system

Help the mind get out of debt and

develop some residual income sources.

There is a life waiting for you with meaning,

intent and peace of mind. Some may have more or
fewer needs, but you know that you can make your
entire life anywhere and under any circumstances.
Someone said, "Life works best for those who make the
most of how life works." Wealth, health, family,
security, beliefs, joy, love and peace of mind are some
of the ingredients in your fulfilment. Your desires, goals,
confidence and passion will play a role in bringing out
everything you deserve. Some of the ingredients were
obtained early in life. Others may take more time. The
time table is uncertain, but it can intensify while you
decide to do what you feel is right for you and others. It
is a divine journey you are on, so you are pleased with
every task as you go through it to your ultimate goal of
achievement.

People can work together to speed up the process and
help you keep track of it. I encourage all of you to take
part in this process, as the bonds contribute to a
stronger force to make the necessary changes in your

life. You can call it rising to a higher consciousness level. We all need to do what we think is right. We are not going to be denied what we rightly deserve. No shortcuts are required for temporary gains. We are looking for a more lasting path that allows us to continue to live better.

Second, you should be very vigilant in protecting your thinking processes. You sometimes confuse yourself with your emotions, so listen to your words and thoughts coming out of your mouth. You get up and down by what's happening in your head. Remember that you are deprived of power, rage, hate, revenge, envy, lust and resentment. In my Discover Living Book, I have said many times that "love makes you like." Stay far from paths leading to mental and physical disorders. Your mind is constantly being exposed to doing, behaving and thinking in ways that try to control or exploit your actions to further others ' aims and not in your best interest.

You are an individual with the right of God to check, question and obey what you feel is right. Your mind should be open to new information, but you need to distinguish right from wrong. A soldier is trained to kill. A baseball player is qualified to hit and hit a baseball. A chef is trained to cook. All these efforts were accomplished by the openness of the mind to new information that brought greater perfection in each particular area of interest. Evaluate the knowledge your brain receives every moment of the day. When the knowledge clashes with any of the above-mentioned four parts of life, decide quickly to discard it in favour of something good that will support your needs and will lead you to a fuller life.

Keep in mind that your emotions are the result of past experiences. To advance in your life, you have to move past emotions, which try to drag you down. Fill your mind with the possibilities for a better future. Miraculous miracles and life changes have happened by filling your mind with the possibilities you are searching for. Relieve yourself from the spinning web of the unpleasant experiences of the past. Your mind is an important link to solving the problems that hold you down in your life. Each one of us is different, so there is no way to lead you to this particular accomplishment you are seeking.

Your needs are private, but the values you want to achieve are common. Start this journey with others. Spread the word for others to join you. Let me repeat myself. Together we become an instrument of experiencing a new level of awareness in which each of us is regarded as a human being and receives the gifts of life that we deserve. Everything is possible. You can start now!

Chapter   3:

How to Increase Your Self-Esteem and Develop Habits

The cutdown definition of self-esteem is one's own positive opinion. The dictionary definition of self-confidence is ability, energy, in some cases, too much.

Although the two are identical, they must work together. They are different. When you look in a mirror and hate the person you see, then your self-esteem is very weak. That's what you ought to focus on. How can you expect others to do this if you don't like and believe in yourself??

Sow a thinking, and you're reaping an act. Sow acting, and you're harvesting the habit. Sow your habit, and you're collecting a character. Habits only repeat the same thing endlessly so that the brain automatically knows what to do. Breathing, heart beating, brain commands for different parts of your body. All these functions are automatic and are completely unconscious. There are, however, other things we can learn to do until they become a habit. It is said that when you play solo, scabbling, crosswords or other brain games with your brain, you build more neural pathways that can slow or stop Alzheimer's disease from occurring. So why don't you use your brain for everything you can. Man uses only about 10% of his brain, normally anyway. This is a higher figure of true geniuses.

Then why don't you train up the neural pathways so that confidence and self-worth will also become an automatic reaction to these qualities? It takes time, of course, if in these areas you are weak, but all good things take time.

Self-esteem bank is the way self-esteem works. You have your own bank account and can only require deposits or cancellations. For example, if someone pays you a compliment, you would automatically allow this deposit to occur. The same occurs if you pay a compliment to yourself. But if someone puts you down, you must put yourself down; then, you have the choice of whether or not to accept it. It's easier to deny someone else a putdown than to withhold it from yourself. You must, therefore, be your own security guard, and you must defend yourself. Consider this a habit too, so that your brain develops another neural path and welcoming compliments, and refusing putdowns is almost another automatic, unconscious function of your mind.

There are three important points about self-esteem.

Firstly, before anyone else does, you must like yourself.

Second, who cares about what others think about you. Your opinion of yourself is very important.

Finally, you can fool some of the people, but you can't fool yourself in the end.

The secret to success is self-confidence and self-esteem.

Progress. You are if you believe you are beaten. If you don't think you dare, you don't. If you want to win but don't think you can, it's almost quartz, you're not going to. If you think you're lost, you lose as you find out in the world, success begins with the will of a man. Everything's in the state of mind. When you think you're out-of-classes, you should think big. Before you ever win a prize, you must be certain of yourself. The fights of life do not always go to the quicker or stronger man. But the one who wins sooner or later is the one who feels he will. Paul Hanna) You're making it the only limit in existence. You have no limitations when you are born. When you grow up, your parents, friends, colleges, universities and employees affect you. You can choose to win or lose. You can achieve as much as you want and part of it is deciding who you can work with. For example, if you are associated with drug users and the criminal element, you are likely to become this kind of person. BUT, you are bound to thrive if you really feel you can when you combine with good, hard-working people in any industry!

You always note, when a person comes into a room, that all eyes seem to be attracted to them when you go to a party or club or even at work. This is because they have a high level of self-confidence and self-esteem and completely believe in themselves. It allows them to radiate their conviction and draw attention. This is a common part of a lot of successful salespeople. All prime ministers. The chairmen and other officials are the same. The. Same. Anthony Robbins is a prime example of a motivational speaker who inspires you with his unlimited passion and radiating self-esteem. You may find your priest, rabbi/reverend, if you go to a place of religious worship, also possesses this mighty sense of self, and this is my absolute faith and devotion to a cause. It's faith in their case. It allows them to radiate their conviction and draw attention. This is a common part of a lot of successful salespeople. All prime ministers. The chairmen and other officials are the same. The. Same. Anthony Robbins is a prime example of a motivational speaker who inspires you with his unlimited passion and radiating self-esteem. You may find your priest, rabbi/reverend, if you go to a place of religious worship, also possesses this mighty sense of self, and this is my absolute faith and devotion to a cause. His faith in this case.

The posture and walking, sitting, standing, and even speaking can be studied to see how various things can be with simple techniques for improving the body and the mind.

NOT EVERYONE FORGETS.

A popular speaker started his seminar with a $20 bill. He asked who would like the $20 note in the space of 200 people. Hands began to arise naturally. He said, "I'm going to give this to one of you, but let me do this first". He crumbled and screwed the note into a ball. Instead, he asked who still wanted it. The hands were up. "Okay", he replied. "What if I do this?" He threw it on the ground and stepped on the note with his shoe on the floor. He took the filthy fucking note. He took it. "Does everyone still want it?" The hands were up. Me and my family have all learned a precious lesson. No matter what I didn't do for the $20, the value didn't decrease. It's still worth 20 cents.

Often in our lives, we are driven down, trampled on, humiliated, and tormented by the decisions we make and the circumstances that come our way. We feel like we're worthless. But whatever happens, you never lose your quality—dry, dusty, crumbled, or fine-tuned. Those who love you are still invaluable. The quality of our lives is not what we do or say, but who we are!

You are different. You are special. Don't ever forget. Don't ever forget. Compare, not your issues, but your blessings. Don't be afraid to try something new.

Some obscure proverbs by writers remember that the amateurs created the ark. The Titanic was designed by professionals.

It was to be it is up to me. It's up to me. So if it's up to me, it must be!

-You can't jump 2 jumps with a chasm!

Believe in yourself. Believe in yourself. For a long time, you must live with yourself to believe more than to admit defeat.

the mind can trust and understand, and it can achieve.

a thousand-mile journey begins with a single step.

-Only if you hesitate to get up again will you struggle.

-Thank you for the issues. This means that you're alive!

Make a list and prioritize your goals. Then concentrate on them one at a time. It is better to do things this way than to stretch yourself too thinly.

Thirteen ways to improve your trust in self-esteem are inside and develop from the inside. So, whenever you want to do something, already imagine yourself there. Take a look and make it true in your heart. Close your eyes and fill out all the specifics-how you would act, how you would comply, how others would comply. So put into action what you see. You think so. You think so.

REACH OUT TO OTHERS

Ask other people nice things. Make a list of what you want and admire in others. If you can, lend a helping hand. We feel more in charge of our own lives by supporting others.

AVOID PERFECTIONISM

Perfectionism paralyzes you and stops you from reaching your goals.

Your physical appearance is a critical factor in your self-esteem. Your physical appearance is a critical factor in your self-esteem. Resist the urge to feel dirty if you feel bad for days. These are really the days when you should be extra careful to look at your best.

GET WITH YOUR OWN CREATIVE ENERGY Get regular practice; you feel more in charge when you can use your body effectively. Listen to music, express art, meditate. Let thoughts come and go as you do these things. Daydream, focus on yourself and concentrate. What were your child's passions? What are you fantasizing about now?

Consideration of YOURSELF. List 50 reasons for your consideration. Think of people who respect and support you and write down what they think about you when you get stuck.

If you are in tough times, seek power and wisdom (Wisdom is Strength, you know) that you wouldn't have if this trauma didn't exist. LOOK ON SILVER LINING.

ACT IN ACCORDANCE

with your own values. Sometimes conflict values. In this scenario, play the role of a friend and discuss the different consequences of each action. Pick what feels best to you.

BE GOOD to YOURSELF ON A DAILY BASIS. Do something that's good for you. Each day!. Every day!

Take a course, CHALLENGE YOURSELF. Travel to a new place–when you are far from a familiar place, it is easier to try out different aspects of your personality. When you face new challenges, you gain new confidence and increase your sense of achievement.

Dispute your cynical ideas. PRACTICE OPTIMISM. Think of misfortunes, rather than permanent and general, as transient and unique. For example,' all managers are jerks' is permanent and omnibus, a view that can lead to a helpless feeling about a particular problem. "He was in a bad mood this morning," is a temporary / specific excuse. This offers hope for improvement.

DON'T TAKE THINGS SO PERSONALLY When someone acts rude or abrasive, he or she shows you something about him or her or how he or she feels right now. Seek to see the pain or fear of the other person from that viewpoint and overcome it.

DON'T TAKE THINGS SO SERIOUSLY

See the moving part of daily calamities. If you see the troubling and amusing side of a given situation, you have a more balanced perspective and approach. Lighten up, lighten up. You will bounce back from disappointments and embarrassing moments quicker, and more people will also like you.

Practice these constructive steps to boost your own self-esteem that will then increase your self-esteem. You will then have the master key for your own performance.

Good Habits Are Easy to Create

Habits-we know all too well the bad habits and the challenge of breaking them. To make a habit, it takes repetition. Everyday life thus becomes a tradition. Life is boring and incredible, and the pressure that affects all of our lives just makes matters worse due to the current economic situation. Everybody experiences the pressure from the oldest family member to the youngest.

Yet, take heart. Such difficult economic times are an opportunity to be innovative, to try to create new ideas and new habits.

Here are five easy tips to help you and your soulmate(s) survive the storm. Say, "I love you," to your soulmate(s) at least once a day. Say that you love them once a day and once a night before going to bed. Hint: "I love you," can also be used all day long: submit generously.

If your kids are not at home anymore, follow the same medication. Get used to messaging them by phone or e-mail twice a day.

Split homemade pizza with a cheap and enjoyable meal which the whole family will contribute to. Most pre-made pizza crusts are available but try the pizza crusts mixture. The easy mix helps you to be imaginative and to make the pizza any shape you can imagine. Seek a heart-shaped pie or butterfly. Crust mix, spaghetti or pizza, mozzarella cheese, pepperoni, or your favourite toppings. Make your family love the tasty, enjoyable, and affordable pizza.

Schedule a regular family time "at home." Rent a movie for the whole family, or rather take a game out of the closet. Hint: The more popular the game is, the more popular it is. Recent findings we enjoyed were "Candyland," "Don't break the ice," and "SORRY."

Limit phone time. We are becoming more attached to our mobiles, and today's communications; technology allows us to spend more and more time in idle conversations. It creates a gap between family members and waste bonding opportunities. We can schedule other times for telephone friends that do not compete with our soulmate(s) time.

Foster creativity in your home. All of us have artistic interests and talents. Discover these passions and strengths in the past, when boredom sets in. Is there an aspiring singer, actress, or family artist? Here are some ideas for fun and creative events that cost little or nothing.

Write a poem or novel.

Sculpt a figurine of clay.

Paint the picture of an aquarelle.

Create a pencil, crayon or pastel design.

Activities that encourage imagination and provide quality time opportunities with our soul mates will reduce stress and strengthen ties. Check these suggestions and find other ways to disrupt the daily routine. Note, by repeating them regularly, you can turn these ideas into good habits.

Some Habits to Live a Healthy Lifestyle

There are many ways to keep your lifestyle commitments healthy; to put a price tag on your failure (bet with someone and be prepared for compensation when you don't follow a plan), set small goals, instead of focusing solely on end results, and find a supportive partner who can help encourage you in the days when you lack motivation.

Seven habits are common for people living in healthy lifestyles. Such patterns are self-mastery and control of our relationships with others and our understanding of the world.

Habit 1: Choose your battle. We're all filled with potentially stressful situations every day, but there is a short time when we are able to choose our special answer from humans. Sadly, all of us have been conditioned in our life to respond to certain situations in certain ways, and we give up our precious right to choose the outcome with conditions of the reaction.

For example, if somebody's rude or offensive, our response will typically be to at least respond with annoyance and sometimes even violence. Instead of embracing this programmed response, we can choose not to allow it to affect us, or even better, to comprehend and forget the stress. If we can have positive or neutral answers, at least, we have the ability to bring us closer to our goals and increase our boundaries. In comparison, poorly selected reactions or programmed reactions that are just unimaginable, would likely have adverse effects and increase our control. This generally leads to an increasingly unregulated feeling of your lot in life as our reactions frequently form our expectations and even evaluate success or failure.

Take responsibility for your health. Poor health and disease are constantly high, and this is a natural part of ageing for many of us. Others accept the burden of their poor health and of their diminished quality of life as something that simply "is" rather than something that can be managed. Instead of becoming involved in self-care, they put themselves in the hands of physicians and pharmaceutical companies. This is a perfect but sad example of a conditioned reaction.

Be positive, challenge the notion that you are a helpless victim instead of embracing poor health and chronic diseases as your destinies, and take responsibility for your wellbeing by cultivating and adopting healthier lifestyles.

Habit 2: Build your' end game' and imagine it.

Get clear about what you really want. Take the time to imagine what it is and whether it's health, more money, a more structured life, or creating a whole new life. Allowing yourself to know exactly what you want in life will help you develop a plan. If this final game is written down or you have built a board where you have cut out images of your ideal life (a dream board), it will enable you to keep it fresh and simple.

Once you have articulated your final game, you will accomplish smaller goals that will eventually help you achieve your desired result. Taking stock of your smaller achievements will allow you to know more about your target. Therefore, having a clear view of your priorities allows you to make smarter decisions that help them.

The wellbeing you have as you grow older will exactly be the culmination of all your health choices until then. If you want to be physically active, mentally sharp and full of energy in your generation, this desired outcome will strongly affect the decisions you make today and every day after.

Poor health or sickness does not occur immediately. While you don't feel as if your health is impaired, chronic inflammatory and acid-forming diets can still encourage your everyday activities, and if they do, it will eventually catch up to you. It can be extremely difficult, but thankfully the damage caused by unhealthy habits can be reversed, and that is why the way you live now should have the best imaginable health decisions, to have a positive effect on your health in your golden years.

Habit 3: Keep your priorities straight. There are only 24 hours a day, and many of the tasks you hope to achieve will not be achieved if you don't handle your time in a wise manner. Mastering the first two behaviours will teach you to take action and become confident about your desired end result, but then you need to have clear understanding and discipline in which to execute actions that help you achieve your objectives. Without that, you will waste time on trivial tasks, and it will become much more difficult to accomplish your goals. Thankfully, you will find that it is easier to stick to your goals by taking small steps to increase productivity (setting timers for activities, uninstalling "Angry Birds" and establishing a concrete plan for the use of Facebook, Twitter and all social networks).

Consider your health your first priority. Many aspects of a healthy lifestyle are often considered restrictive, time-consuming, or simply challenging. When you try to follow too restrictive and complicated lifestyles, you will definitely get brutalized and irritated, and you will most likely return earlier than later to your old unhealthy practices. But that can not be prevented when, instead of taking away negative aspects of your habits, you spend your time and effort wisely by focusing on contributing to healthy activities and food. The better would eventually crowd out the bad.

Let's assume, for starters, that you hate the gym. You decide to start a healthy lifestyle so you can register for a gym. You go and buy shoes, clothing, all the bells and whistles that the gym entails. You go for a week, two, perhaps even a few months. You slowly learn that you don't like running on a treadmill, you can't stand waiting for weight machines, you can't jockey for Zumba school. You decrease your time in the gym, first by 10 minutes and then by one day and before you know it, that one day becomes a long time. If what you really like doing is being outside, instead of going to the gym, take a 20-minute walk away before or after dinner and choose a spot you prefer. If you like shopping, going window shopping is a great way to learn what you are going to buy by saving the pound. You sit at a desk all day, so why not build a standing workspace and pick up a pedal bike. Creating 5-minute breaks every 20 minutes of work, touching your knees, picking up kids ' shoes, moving your car away from the mall and taking your three-way stairs up to your apartment instead of the elevator are great ways to exercise. If you do this every day, going to the gym won't be necessary.

With meat, instead of using cold turkey on all your favourite foods, you might want to choose to incorporate spinach rather than Roman salad in your wraps. Try a new fruit or vegetable. In a week, you agree to a meatless meal. Then you begin to notice that you become happier with foods that don't have as much space as you would for junk food usually. There are many ways to make your food savoury, so you never feel deprived. Healthiness must not be painful.

Habit 4: Win scenario/Cultivate. All of us use personal gain instinctively as a strong motif in life. Due to this fact, most of the issues or challenges facing others are best solved with a solution that benefits everyone.

Most people are only worried about "what is there for them" and pay little attention to the impact of their actions on others. Many people limit themselves, often without understanding, because without the help and support of others, it is much more difficult to achieve goals. Also unlikely in some situations. Ever since they do know in time that they need support from those around them, they are unlikely to get it because they appear to be self-centred and oppressive.

Seek a win with your health. Often it takes a great deal of discipline and determination to maintain and retain good health due to the many disruptive and negative influences of our culture. The support of the people around you makes it much easier. With this in mind, when you enable your healthy lifestyle to impact other people's lives, you will find that they resist change in your healthy lifestyle or risk alienating others, which makes it more difficult to adopt a healthy lifestyle.

Your family members appear to be your most important partnerships and have the greatest support capacity, and it is important that they are on your side. Better health is a clear win for yourself, but your attempts to do so can be a source of controversy among your family members. Your goals for better health, though, could also be a big win for your family if you handle the situation intelligently.

Habit 5: To understand suffering and to not at least recognize the point of view of other people is the number one explanation why many ties erode.

It is often natural to drive your opinion further when someone contradicts an opinion that you hold strongly. This often faces other challenges and can trigger a downward spiral that leads to a hideous argument or even a broken relationship. The only way to avoid this situation and turn it into a constructive conversation is to make a strong effort to understand the opposite viewpoint before you speak against it. Whether you realize that the resistance is based on a misunderstanding in many situations, you will learn something new.

In search of better health, it is a virtual certainty that you will hear several different points of view and ideas, also from doctors and health workers. Most views would contradict each other diametrically. Big business ' revenues continue to exacerbate these different perspectives, sometimes creating more uncertainty with every new dietary book that is written. Health-related views are often debated intensely, and, as such, the need for active and considerate interaction increases significantly.

Habit 6: Synergy harmonization also results from the two previous behaviours. When all parties focus on finding a solution for everyone, and when all different opinions are taken into consideration, the result is usually a variety of imaginative ideas and possibilities that would never have been individually conceived.

The human body is a complex organism, and many questions still remain unanswered by modern medicine. As a consequence, some health conditions can seem unresolvable. A one-sided approach to any health condition is never as successful as the synergistic approach to treating the disease. Through listening to the different views shared through medical professionals, physicians, families and friends, we also open the door for new ideas and possibilities to strengthen and even renew our well-being.

Habit 7: Stay sharp, concentrated, and balanced. Being productive will intentionally advance towards a set target. The past six habits provide the resources you need to help stability and growth in the physical, emotional, mental, and social aspects of your life and become a fuller and more productive person. Staying fresh and concentrated means keeping the development on track.

Keeping our bodies safe is important for our ability to fully enjoy life. To be spiritually confident and having a firm understanding of our beliefs and inspirations helps us to lead our lives to what we want to experience. Staying mentally sharp and developing our awareness strengthens our ability to understand and accept our faith and maintain our lives along the way. Eventually, social interaction is one of the most rewarding aspects of life, offering us a sense of belonging, fulfilling and encouraging better health in exchange.

Chapter 4: How to Break Bad Thinking Habits

I am surprised that people really believe they live with true freedom of choice. I know this is a comment that could and will make many of you uncomfortable. Of course, every day, you have the right to decide which religion to practice or for whom you choose to vote in the presidential elections. After all, we who live in the United States respect the principle of freedom and the ability to live a life of freedom and happiness. While our Constitution can grant us such rights, we are more enslaved than we wish to admit, as individuals. Science shows how connected we are to our subconscious behaviour, behaviours and habits.

Many habits work well here, like teeth being brushed, toilets being used if we need to and thanking people are kind to us. Certain habits such as eating, using tobacco, or alcohol are too easily driven to rage and quickly susceptible to desperation are behaviours that do not support our health. Neuroscience research reports that 40-90% of our day-to-day practices are carried out unconsciously. (Do you remember what happened when you went to work today?) We survive on pre-installed software that has been learned from our experience for a long time.

With practical MRIs, PET scans and other tools, our ability to understand how the brains work is enhanced. The study of habit creation in major universities and think tanks is booming. The idea is that if we understand how our brain creates subconscious patterns, we can learn to create new patterns that benefit our health, well-being, and, hopefully, also our planet's.

In his novel, The Power of Habit, Charles Duhigg writes in great depth, explaining three aspects of the "habit-loop." The signal is the catalyst in our setting, which knows that we want something and that it activates a well-tried and automatic behaviour that leads us to some kind of reward. The theory is basic training on Madison Avenue, where we know how to create a desire that is the hallmark. Once this circuit in our brain is well known as a normal neural loop, it remains there effortlessly. There is some evidence that a pattern never really goes away. Once it is established, it is only locked in, resulting in a more powerful reward. One example could be to see a happy couple (cue) that is followed by a lonely feeling that leads to a journey to an ice cream dessert freezer (routine), personal favourite Haagen Dazs chocolate chip pint (reward).

The notion that patterns never really disappears, they are forever embedded in the brain's anatomy, that can be rather upsetting. However, it is important to understand that certain habits are critical to survival and allow the brain to achieve energy saving. Through creating new software that works as well as a CD boot when you plug it into the CD drive on your device, behaviours place less on energy reserves of the brain. It takes more energy than to repeat a known series of events to experience something new. Habits can be described as the decisions that we made with deliberation, which were analytical, automatic and repeated in the same way, time after time. The ability to customize and choose what we want to create and maintain and which we need to prune is a critical and masterful ability to develop.

The minds don't really distinguish good and bad habits, they work equally well in both kinds collectively. One could claim that the sanctuary that comprises the characteristics of wisdom is our brain. Therefore, the mind does not really know what is going on in our external environment or in our inner thoughts. Does your belief system question this? There are numerous studies that have essentially shown that the cable of the brain reacts just as much to the real thing as to the real thing. For example, playing a piano Brahms concert stimulates the same neurons as when one thinks of playing the same notes. The area of sports training uses this method to train world-class athletes psychologically all the time.

I advise you to read and discuss Dr Joe Dispenza's research. His first novel, Evolving Your Mind, and his most recent book, Breaking Your Self Habit: how to lose your mind and create a new one. I had the opportunity recently to spend some weekends with him. He explains in his books and workshops that when we encounter something new, certain thoughts and feelings are created. These thoughts and feelings become our recollections forever, particularly when an emotion was involved and related to them rather than a neutral event or observation. If the memory creates a particular feeling in the mind, say guilt. For example, this contributes to other unpleasant remorseful thoughts and memories that create a neurotransmitter that signals the body to create those emotions that are transmitted back to the brain and the cycle goes on indefinitely. This cycle allows our cell receptors to get used to and addicted to these chemicals, which then leads the cells to feel satisfied by higher doses or fixes. One could then presume that as individuals, we will generate more and more life experiences that are in line with the need to repair our cells. This is how our history is our future crystal ball.

"If you think of your past memories, you can only construct previous experiences." So when we try to remove old habits and develop healthy new ones, like walking rather than watching American Idol and eating kale chips instead of potato chips, we should create a different new state of mind from the old. Research also shows that the positive reversal of what is considered a keystone habit greatly empowers us to bring about further improvements by concentrating on modifying a pattern.

While it is our propensity to behave robotically and predictably, we do not have such a life as a living version of Groundhog Day. Remember when I said that the brain wiring does not know the difference between what occurs internally and externally? This can be an enormous benefit. We may build a neural net by consciously rehearsing new behaviours and patterns that will become stronger once it is rethought. The processing of a new piece of information was shown to build up to 2600 new brain synapse connections. A new thought by concentrating on a new way of doing something that is reinforced by the repetition of thought, mental seeing and feeling (feelings are the way the body knows and they are completely an integral part of the process), is a way that can create a new and better mechanism for the creation of a new pattern habit. When the new road becomes more enticing than the old custom, which generates new and safer benefits, the older habit is submerged and a new way of being can emerge.

It is, therefore, possible, if it is your wish, to have a healthier body, create a stronger and more intimate relationship, or grow into a more purposeful vocation. As I said, be prepared to put as much effort into creating a new way of being as you were able to do in order to create an old way.

Be Serious About Your Goals

Staying Firm With Your Life Goals

Be careful about your goals. You haven't got time to waste.

You only need to lose your life literally if you want to succeed in life. Most of you walk through life without reason, without a focus, without a goal. It's not you when doing that.

You are different. You were different.

The reason why you are reading this chapter in this book is because you want a better life for yourself, or perhaps want to change yourself, your family, your car, or your home.

You are sure you are ready to change and will do whatever you can to make this happen.

You want to change things; you want to get better things for yourself because you're sick of being unhappy. You're dissatisfied with something that's unjust, tiring, dull, stunting, and furious.

You want to change things.

I know that's you; the first thing you have to do is stop complaining when you've taken it as a joke.

You should examine yourself if you don't live the life you deserve. Perhaps you took your career unfavourably. Looking around you, you see that you have no concentration, intent, or sight.

Yet one thing I know about you is that it's not you. You need stuff to change and stuff to develop. You're prepared to change things because you're sick of a circus and you're the clown.

It is time for you to live a stable, healthy, peaceful life you really deserve.

It's you. You must be ready to accept that your life, your hopes and your dreams are no longer a joke.

When you take what you're about and what you want to do seriously, everyone else will support and appreciate you because you're serious about who you are and where you want to be. Gain your respect and recognition.

Objectives are not drawn to clowns; they are attracted to the people who have chosen the brightest, the best and the extreme.

To be happy, calm, positive and successful in life, it is a matter of self-dialogue that you listen to or speak to yourself. Adjust it, and life will change. Self-dialogues are amazing and powerful when you trust them.

Begin with this: Your vision will make you tremble so vividly in your body that you are persuaded, that the purpose of your life is what you are doing. It gives you the confidence you need in life, no doubt about it.

You should know what you want, be sure of what you need and be certain that it belongs to you as you go through your life. You deserve it. You deserve it. That's all you can say to yourself every day.

And as you do these things, you must always remember to tell yourself that there is no space in your mind for negative things like anxiety, doubt or abandonment. You don't have to poison your brain.

Your only thoughts should be suggestions which will get you where you want to be. You have a vision to fulfil, a desire to accomplish, and a need to change your life. This is your only priority, nothing else.

Note that we haven't got time to waste. Life is no longer a joke. We only need to stop wasting our precious resources in thoughts that won't allow us to rise.

We are special, differentiate yourself from the rest.

You are different. You are different. Your feelings ought to be too. Only those who accomplish life's goals are those who choose to differ from others. They're the ones where fear doesn't exist because they think differently. Your thinking has changed differently and even Mutated.

Only through feeding thoughts, ideas and pictures will you be able to construct a broad repository of self-growth ideas.

Ask yourself, "What ideas do I need to help myself grow?" Do not accept mediocrity any longer. This is a feeling in your mind that you have to believe and carve.

What do you have in common with successful individuals? It is the capacity to assume that we deserve more than mediocrity.

Let me clarify, you have to train your mind to believe that most successful people enjoy themselves because they accept their problems and have chosen to do something about them, dissatisfied with a certain portion of their lives. You chose not to accept your low-paid job anymore because you knew that you wouldn't get anywhere if you kept it. Step away from toxic ties, change your jalopy. Change yourself.

They changed it. It changed. We are the kind of people who can no longer tolerate mediocrity. You must do this too.

You're upset with life because it's not normal. This resentment is against you for not taking the initiative. You have to be ready to do something, fight for it, do what you have to do. Nothing, I presume! Do something at least, even if you look like a fool.

What will inspire you to act is to believe that you are brought to life on this earth?

You need to know your love life.

Things are going to change.

Motivate yourself to follow your dreams, your ambitions and to enjoy the possibilities that life offers you. Those who want to love life will be changed.

It's you.

If your mind is changed, you won't settle for mediocrity anymore. You have chosen to be special. Don't console yourself with a bad and miserable life. Adjust now. Improve now.

Start today.

When you have had enough, when you're going to change, once you open your eyes, you see how much and more you deserve to live. It is the turning point in your life when you know you are different, you want more out of life, and it is time to live the life that you deserve. It starts with being a new you, a fresh start.

You have to build thoughts and believe in them to finish this. You deserve them. You deserve them. Trust in them. Believe in them. You're more valuable than you think. If you change your way of thinking, you will thank yourself.

Give yourself suggestions and things that make you happy.

How To Realize Your Life Goals

It's not as difficult to find your life goal when you take this step; you have to decide your true value, you should remove any obstructions that hold you. You should achieve a life goal which enables you to pursue your interests while still supplying you with basic necessities of life. You should eventually put your life in order and take action.

How do we discover our true values? Well, you can start by working through various aspects of your life to figuring out what each one of them is about.

Examples include: at the workshop, exercising at the gym, having lunch with friends, playing tennis, going to the movies, walking the dog, doing a college job, mowing the lawn. You should choose a combination of activities that include things you really want to do and at least a few things you do because you need to. For each of these things, write down everything that you think about immediately.

If you have done that to each of them, sit back and try commonalities and topics. Through careful thoughts and an open mind, you will begin to realize what you really like, what is important, and what is not.

Your life goal is most probably activities that reflect on your core values, and it is up to you to decide exactly what these activities are going to be. Next, you need to figure out what keeps you from doing fun things and what you can do to improve this.

Blocks can take many forms, just like when you are too lazy to get out of the lounge and do stuff. Or it could be more troublesome, as another one actually stops you from doing things you love (possibly because of a conflict of values). Blockages can also be more complex than the culture of which you belong and do not accept certain aspects of your activities, and you would have to break all relationships to pursue your dreams.

More insidious obstacles can also occur, such as two values in which you truly treasure conflict with each other, so you do nothing. Whatever kind of blockage you have, it is important to eliminate or at least find workable compromises before you actually set a life goal.

The successful setting of a life goal is an extremely satisfying thing to do, and the key is "successful." You would need to decide what sort of time you will spend on your life goal, will this be a full or part-time commitment? If you are willing to follow your passion in the full time, you should make sure that you have the income to live on, whether investments or income that you can benefit directly from your new effort.

Faced with the facts, many people are pursuing their new goal with a focus on just running out of money sometimes. It is far better to plan finances beforehand and to know the most likely scenarios for what is next.

When you only plan to start with a part-time dedication now, you can continue to earn revenue from an alternative activity. It is now up to you, with this kind of realistic plan in place, to evaluate your entire life and reassess everything in which you are involved and set your goals for the greatest possible outcome.

The best bit of advice is to treat the key things that you do in your life as urgent / not urgent and important. After you have done this, you can classify these important things into a quadrant. The Quadrants are: urgent / important; important / not urgent; not important / urgent.

The obvious thing to do is focus your attention as much as possible on what is urgent and important and cut out as many things that are not important / not urgent as possible. Items that are relevant and not urgent should be considered your second priority. This is a simple talent to structure your goals in this way, but once you do, you will profit abundantly.

Creating a life goal isn't something to be taken lightly, but it will also give you immense joy if you do it correctly. If you use the above-mentioned measures, it will certainly help you in your studies, but it is important to note that there is a lot to learn about this subject and it is important to do more research to develop your knowledge. As with all significant "transform" work, the action is necessary, and momentum is created. You, too, can create a magical life! Carpe diem (seize the day).

Chapter 5: Life Happiness Depends on Your Life Goal

People don't know what course is better for them. They don't know what shirt or clothes to choose from. They don't even know what to eat for lunch. Everyone likes to ask for a different opinion about their own question. Yet their life continues to repeat all this without worrying about solving them. Why do people find it hard to make a simple decision? Do people think life is hard for an ordinary human being?

Actually, life is very easy. It all depends on your purpose in life. If you don't have a goal for life or don't have a clear idea about your goals in life, your life isn't simple anymore. You are not sure about your life goal if you don't know which path is right for you. If you are asking other people for advice in your own life (not relating to knowledge), you are not sure about your life purpose.

I firmly believe you should tell yourself what your life goal is when you don't know which shirt you should wear one day. If you're upset with someone, tell yourself what your life goal is. If you are concerned about the outcome of your test, you must tell yourself what your life goal is. We ought to be responsible for our own emotions. You should tell yourself what is wrong with you if you find you are in a kind of emotion that you don't like. Isn't your life goal all right? And, even worse, you have no clear objective.

Why can we allow another issue to occur? Why don't we try to solve it for once in our life? Do we assume that the issue is usual for an ordinary person? Do we think life is packed with many unfortunate events/things? We don't seem to be responsible for our feelings.

If we have set our life goal, we should be responsible for all its consequences, including our anger. If we can't accept these effects, we're expected to change the goal.

The target could make our lives exciting. The target could always make us fail. The target will make our life simple and happy. What kind of life depends on your purpose? Please do not blame people for being sad. It's really ridiculous to ask for advice on our own life. Why could people help if they don't know your life goal, and you only know it yourself? Someone even offers guidance on their own purpose in life rather than yours. They thought you should also use the same approach when you solve the problem.

Let's say you're going to choose a university education, and there's course A and course B ahead. If you choose course A, are you going to reach your goal? Please ask yourself. If you choose course B, can you follow your objective? If both courses allow you to achieve your goal, choose one. If you just take Class A to achieve your goal, choose Class A. If you can not achieve your goal in both courses, you must find the course that helps you achieve it. What's so hard? The hard part is if we have no life goal. If that is the case, no one can rescue you. You can't ask someone how the problem can be solved. You are the nature of the problem. It's not from the setting. There are, of course, some people who solve the problem through another process. You try to find out which course will be more popular or which course will give you more money in the future. You no longer have this kind of concern (internal factor). It's an outside factor. If you have incorrect information, notice it and feel angry about it after you enter the course, what triggers your anger? It is caused by you, not by the person who gave you the data. When choosing your course using this type of process, you should be mindful of this type of risk and consider all the consequences.

Happiness is personal. Happiness is personal. So we should do whatever we do, make whatever choices, and not let anyone do this for us. We must base our decision on what we want for our lives. We can't let others decide (just my suggestion) our happiness. When you allow others to decide for you, you have to accept the consequences and be content with everything you face. It's difficult to find someone who allows others to control their lives and still feel very happy with their lives.

The primary factor in differentiating adults with children is that adults can take responsibility and know the consequences very well, but children can't. When we look around, we can find many people with an adult body who cannot take responsibility for the consequences and do not know or care about it. You can't be responsible for their own emotions in general. In reality, our emotion is the product of our decision.

Our goal of life is our option. We should think deeply about achieving our best goal. We have 100% control to choose our own life goal based on our purpose and what we want. After the target has been determined, we work for our goal. Everything that happens after that affects our emotions. Emotion is, therefore, the product of our purpose in life. Emotion is our own option. Emotion.

Present steps determine future results.

We are already aware of the importance of self-discipline, but do we need it?

We know about performance methods, and we know a lot of useful resources that lead to success, so why do we need self-discipline?

For many areas of our lives, we all have goals. Some of us want good ties, others want more money, some want joy in their lives, and others want a better health with less weight. This goal sometimes fails to be achieved. The common question is: Why do we not meet these objectives? Why don't they excel in these objectives?

The overall response is lack of self-discipline.

Success requires time. It doesn't happen immediately. What you do today will determine your future results. When you change your present, the future will change. You will gain weight by eating several pizzas and delicious foods today, and this will be shown in your future weight. You will have less money in the future if you spend more money than you earn now.

Present actions determine future outcomes.

Self-discipline takes place in your present, leading to your future.

You can learn some ideas and strategies for your goals, but if you do not take action to reach them, you will never succeed. Nearly all objectives require effort and continuity. Self-discipline helps you make the requisite commitments and consistency. If you need to lose weight, you need to have less self-discipline. If you want to make more money, you should make more savings or more investments. Self-discipline takes time and performance.

It's all about giving. Sure, this means making some tough compromises often. Why do we need to sacrifice? Why not just enjoy the time and do what we want to do?

Obviously, nobody will pressure you to do anything that you really don't want to do. We compromise, however, because we have ideals and essential goals in our lives and these values allow us to choose whether it is fun or not. In most instances, the two can not be done at the same time.

Our lives are filled with temptations: TVs, good food, chocolates, video games... and so on. It is hard for us to avoid having more fun, and therefore we ignore the most important goals of our lives. Nearly all of us want a slim figure, but we lose this aim of a slim figure with these temptations nearly always around us. Nearly all of us want to make more money, but resistance to discounted travel packages isn't easy, for example. We need self-discipline in these matters. These allow us to focus on and follow our goals before we succeed. Through self-discipline, we can manage our immediate desires better.

There is a difference between what you think and what you know.

It's the limit of your heart and brain.

It's an incredible resource for performance. In reality, most experts believe that success without it is unlikely. "Success is impossible, period," says Lou Holtz. Research shows that entrepreneurs must do this to succeed in business. He found that what was popular among successful men is not their education or intellect or learning, but their high self-discipline, according to Jerry Oster young, which worked with 3,000 people. Studies show that high school success is linked instead of high IQ rates to high self-discipline. I encountered a student aged 21 who completed his high school with straight A's. For just one year he went to medical school and dropped out. He didn't finish his studies. He also declined coaching or treatment. At 154, his IQ score was extremely high. He certainly did not need coaching to learn with his high intelligence. Nonetheless, he definitely needed coaching to learn. He simply did not want to learn, and despite his intellect, he did not complete his studies. There was no training for himself to learn.

It is the tradition of successful people.

It's a habit of the brain.

Successful people are psychologically conditioned for self-discipline. They use it automatically and naturally. It ensures that they don't have to produce and use it daily.

We recognize that there is a pattern and common law of progress. We also know that successful people have only succeeded in implementing these rules. Several scholars have long researched successful people and have written several rich and valuable books about them. One of the world's top experts, Brian Tracy, says that the ability of self-discipline is a key skill to achieve success. You may know some achievements laws, and you may have a strategy for your goals, but if you do not exercise self-control for your objectives, this map will not work. 97% of people don't write their goals, which alone is a huge barrier to success, but it's not enough to write their goals simply unless it is paired with self-discipline. It's your realistic progress chart. Your pragmatic steps are the ones that lead you to the success of your goals.

Successful people have high self-discipline and use it without difficulty. We do not see it as a tough sacrifice or boring mission, but rather as a kind of independence. Free reliance on others, free retreat and freedom from self-limitation.

For all areas of our lives, we need it. It is linked to the skills of time management. With it, you can organize your time better. It can lead to self-esteem, independence and self-satisfaction. You will also need it for spiritual growth, self-growth and meditation.

It's one of the key tools to do what you can, your potential.

Some people were born with high discipline. Nonetheless, the majority of people don't have it, and they can know it. This training can take two forms: by conscious methods, i.e. routine activities for some time, a month or so. Or through subconscious devices like hypnosis, which is more powerful and enduring. In either way, the person can acquire self-discipline and complete the tasks required.

Be mindful of Distracting Urges.

One of the principles of personal development is to change behaviour. You need to change your behaviour to a certain degree if you want to develop yourself.

It doesn't actually rework itself, but it's still a shift.

The whole reason for changing yourself is to change what you are. Many things don't work for you, because the action you need is absent.

Or you just want to make things better. And to do that, you need new skills. Changing actions can also involve learning new skills.

Once you learn new skills and apply new skills, there is an improvement in attitude, and you take advantage of the new skills.

So how's one attitude changing? The capacity for self-discipline is at the root of changing behaviour. This is also regarded as self-control and self-will.

You can have all the world's knowledge. Nevertheless, if you have no freedom to integrate this information into your actions, knowledge is of no use.

You know, for starters, that you should not do certain things. But what is the point of knowledge if you do those things anyway?

Personal development experts will tell you this: you should set goals and split tasks into sub-tasks, prioritize tasks and write newspapers.

But if you have no self-discipline to apply all of this advice, you're not going to succeed! And it can lead you to blame for the failure of expert advice.

Nevertheless, what is self-discipline? It's the eternal struggle between the two. We always have a self that is mindful of long-term objectives. We get and remember what's right for us.

Then we get the other, hyperactive and hedonistic self. This other person is always drawn to the culpable pleasures they should not pursue. This other person is the one that prevents us from taking the initiative that we should take.

The driving self needs a sweet treat, is faint-hearted and just brings to watching TV. The better person knows that these are bad things. And in particular, you really should sleep healthy, exercise and focus on making that phone call.

The impulsive self on the deeper level is a primal self, impulsive, looking for and desiring things. The better ones are our theoretical ones. This is the neo-cortex that functions. It is the recent part of our brain that plays a complex role. That part of the brain has a large picture, balances different choices and knows what's right and wrong.

Who doesn't want success, good relations, an excellent-being and health? Who doesn't want to be glad? All this can be accomplished by full independence.

The fundamental reasons many people fail to practice self-control and give in to the impulsive self are the fact that they don't even excel after reading books, taking courses or attend seminars.

The root of all personal problems lies in the discipline's failure. The underlying reason people can't succeed is because they can't remain self-disciplined.

Self-discipline is the greatest strength of mankind.

You may wonder if self-discipline can be increased.

And the answer is a resounding YES.

One can definitely increase the willpower he or she has.

Power is a commodity of minimal value. In other words, self-discipline is gaining ground. Even after self-discipline, your willpower will be weakened, and you don't do that well if you have to exercise your willpower.

But if you continue to practice self-discipline, it improves. It could sound counterintuitive. They just said that the use of willpower makes it worse, but they suggest that the use of its time and again strengthens it.

The best analogy is that of the body. The muscle is exhausted and sore right after the use. But if you continue to practice, again and again, your muscle strength and tone will increase.

When you practice self-discipline consciously over and over, you will improve it. You will increase the level of self-discipline.

What are the ways to improve the strength of will?

The last decade of study in human psychology has shown many ways in which the will or self-discipline can be strengthened. Kelly McGonigal, a Stanford psychologist, discusses four ways to improve willpower.

Get enough rest. Get enough sleep.

Less sleep is one of the most important ways to improve willpower.

In reality, lack of sleep prevents us from functioning at most. If we are deprived of sleep, our prefrontal cortex does not work much, which means that our defensive mind is not involved and we are quick to cede.

It's important to sleep well at night. This takes 7 hours for most people. If you haven't slept for 7 hours and don't feel sleepy, the cortex doesn't work fully. It is therefore very necessary to sleep for 7 hours.

Meditation is one of the methods that can be used successfully to help you get more sleep.

Forgive yourself. Forgive yourself.

Generally, we condemn ourselves. We tend to criticize us, especially when we have a setback.

Scientists found that for reasons we do not fully understand, we tend to repeat such a loss or indulgent conduct when we are critical of ourselves or when we are stern about reticence.

On the other hand, if you forgive yourself for retrogression, it seems to prevent future retrogressions.

So learn to forgive yourself for your journey's setbacks.

Pay attention to irritating impulses.

Awareness of your desires and impulses is one of the most important tools to improve self-discipline.

It becomes easier not to react if you can develop the conscious awareness of irritating urges.

You need to remember that when you meet a distracting desire or anxiety, it will ruin your target.

We experience various kinds of impulses. You may feel like you're stuck, and you're not going to start reading the book. Or you might want to delay that important class registration. You can feel the temptation to indulge in high-calorie food if your aim is to lose weight.

What you do here. Here is what you do.

Note the way that you feel. Take note of the thoughts that pass through your mind. Note the momentum. Feel the pain.

Be aware of the momentum. Feel the energy, what is this? What is it? What's the sensation? Where's the sensation? Is it somewhere in the body?

Take part in this inner experience. Recognize the feeling and embrace it. Seek not to avoid the feeling. Face it and accept it.

Take a deep breath and pause when acknowledged. Give your body an opportunity to slow down and prepare.

Once you have experienced the inner experience closely, bring your attention to your target. Consider behaviour that will help you achieve your objective.

In fact, this is your desire or motivation, then it embraces it and goes on to what is right to do.

This can be better for meat pulses. It is more difficult to know the habit of postponing stuff. But you can strengthen by training.

Visualize blocks of roads.

People usually think you have to envision success to be a success. Run the self-help guru from the factory that would say that you have to imagine success and not failure.

Yet comprehensive research indicates that predicting success alone is inadequate. Sure, it's a good idea to envision success. But a better idea is to imagine failure regularly! You may think that will lead you to failure, but that's not what happens in practice.

Two groups of people were compared in one scientific study. One team also visualized the final targets. They visualized the end goal.

Another team visualized the end goal and the process of making the path to success. The visualized ups and downs of the process reflect the success and improvements they made along the journey.

The team that also visualized the trip was double the chance of achieving the actual results.

The path to reach the goal is, therefore, more important than the goal itself.

What will you inevitably face during the journey? There are many failures. And the losses would demoralize you for a weak heart and cause you to abandon your target. There won't only be one loss, but many of them.

Failure's unavoidable. So you brace failure to imagine failure. Despite having visualized failure repeatedly with success, it's no longer a surprise when you're actually hit by failure. You're up for it already.

So imagine the trip every day and envision a loss.

Allow your future family.

Usually, we don't worry much about what will happen to us in the future. We don't visualize our own future. Our understanding of our future self might seem to be very powerful in terms of willpower.

When you think of your future self as being completely different from your present self, i.e. when you dissociate your present self entirely from your future self, the future self is like a stranger, and you don't know much about the future self.

In such situations, you don't bother to look after yourself, because your future self is a stranger for all practical purposes.

Different people have different views of themselves in the future. Many people think of them as their present self. Most assume that their future selves are very different.

The desire to withdraw from the long-term effects of your decisions makes you impulsive. Even where options are not important to future implications.

In these situations, you are less open to your future worries and plans. In fact, we know that we have to look after our future self. We must save up for retirement and look after our children by planning for our future.

The question is, how can we bind our future self more? A useful method, used primarily by scientists, is letter writing. Write your present self a letter from your future self.

Or you can write to yourself, remember who you are and what is happening in your life. Chronicle the challenges today. To address yourself from your future to your present self.

The aim is to communicate via communication with your future self. It is better to be hopeful in your letter to the future than to be cynical.

This exercise is not intended to look at this phase as if you are setting things for your future self. It's more about knowing that your future self is true and will be you.

This isn't so much that you are going to be the same person.

Even if you begin to imagine doing worldly things in the future. Like driving to work, shopping and talking to friends, or doing homework. Picture exactly what it will be like for several years.

Here's the rundown.

Self-discipline is the greatest strength of the human being.

One of the main reasons for this loss is the lack of self-discipline.

Power of will may be increased.

Sleep well. Sleep well.

Forgive yourself. Practice forgiveness.

Cultivate knowledge of your triggers and urges.

Visualize gaps and faults of roads.

Practice linking yourself in the future.

Chapter 6: Procrastination Is Your Enemy

Who and what you are now is only the product of your positive behaviour. The same goes for what you are going to be as a man. Getting caught up in the destructive habit of procrastination can only immobilize you and rob you of a future that may be a fantasy. Overcoming delay has no magic "cure" but allows you to really build and increase your capacity to act. Procrastination is a truly odd behaviour, but it's certainly there by design, as it gives you the requisite resistance to drive you on in order to build your inner strength and your "emotional muscle." Procrastination allows you to postpone the activities that will bring you the results that you aim to achieve. You must step up and reinforce your resolve. The easiest way to get involved is to make a decision. Decision is the father of action and all action is determined. The problem is that we have used the word judgment so broadly that it has lost much of its true significance. When you make a real decision, a real choice, you cut off all other options than what you are completely committed to. Like any other talent, you need to enhance decision-making by taking more of them and as you grow this ability, you can increase your progress before you finally develop a decisive habit.

A truly dedicated choice will turn the' should' into' musts,' which distinguishes procrastinators from definitive achievements. We get what we need and our' must' only when it's convenient. The most common reason people do not feel like doing this is because they don't like it. If you don't like to do it, it just means that you combine more pain with action than to avoid it. As human beings, our emotions and feelings are largely controlled. You're going to do virtually anything to avoid painful emotions and pleasure. Your belief in what will lead to pain or pleasure serves as a reference for decision-making. Changing your restrictive beliefs is a powerful way to overcome delays. The only reason you can't act is due to your belief(s) that you can't.

Beliefs are designed to make decisions quickly as a short cut for your mind. Even if you do not have accurate experiences, your mind will build on your beliefs. We all need certainty, and our faith gives us that sense of certainty. The most powerful beliefs of all are your beliefs and your own abilities. If you believe that you are a doctrine and that you can never follow up and produce results, you will always be a doctrine regardless of what technique or strategy you learn or apply. Your belief in you creates your identity and one of your character's strongest need is to ensure that your actions are consistent with your identity. Whatever identity you have, your reality will be created.

Your convictions are mainly unconsciously formed by life experiences and the meaning. You are the master of meaning and the way you express your impressions to yourself defines the importance of things to you. The way you talk and communicate with yourself is a form of hypnoses, and most people are having real trouble screwing. They have a negative conversation about themselves. This creates powerless beliefs about their capabilities. To overcome the delay, you have to take control of your internal communication. What you think about yourself and your life will finally decide what you do.

People who are happy, successful and satisfied are not perfect or born under the right stars, but individuals are those who have learned how to conquer and behave even if they don't feel like it. You really aren't in a resourceful emotional state when you don't feel like doing it. The easiest way to change this is to change your mind; change your focus and what you take care of. You will eventually start to hesitate if your focus is on the frustrating and negative aspects of any mission, even if you are extremely disciplined. Your focus is on your life experience. Learning to control and concentrate yourself on the enjoyable aspects of action will help you to overcome discomfort. Build the habit of looking at the result and not the process and watch yourself go past decline.

Steps to Having Achievable Objectives

Build your next scene and follow these tips. An experienced archer watches the target 25 meters away. The bow in his hand is taken, the rope is extended, the arrow is directed towards the target and hit. In this sequence, we set the goal as the archer's "goal" and the goal as the direction that the arrow traces to the goal. How many objectives are needed to achieve the objective here? In the moment when the archer set the target, it led to many possibilities that he would achieve. The wind in the scenario, the weight and type of arrow used, the power done in the ark at the time of the shot, the distance between the target and it, the position in the body to carry out the launch; eventually he achieved his goal because he had the ability to evaluate all his practice variables and was prepared to conquer them all.

For example, when deciding to make money online, we have to create those objectives, including creating a website, fashion, connections with customers that intellectually inspire you in the field of digital marketing, etc. Do you understand? Do you understand? Various goals could lead us to one goal. Explaining that, let us now define some variables to consider when setting goals:

1-Make your goal specific. Your goal should be well established. It's useless to say that you want to purchase a house. Defining which type of home you want, how many rooms you should have, what attracts you in and out, the place, the price you are prepared to pay if you want a garage. The more your target is established, the more you will be guided.

2-An aim must be attainable, feasible and achievable. Do not use looking for homes that are valued above its pre-established objective, because it becomes lord and frustrates your achievement.

3–Objectives should be challenging and important. To achieve the goal, it takes courage. Many in life do not accomplish goals just because they have no confidence to hazard. Test and error are taught and accomplished. So, take up the challenge and follow your goals. Remember: "While good is expected, good is not good"-Tom Rabbit.

4-Make an action plan. Your ability to set goals and prepare their accomplishment is the "basic ability" for success. The aim of the planning is to allow you to achieve your main objective more easily and with less obstacles. Make a multi-way model with well-defined stages-start, medium and end-set deadlines and sub-periods. Make a plan to build goals for each goal.

5–Achieve existing obstacles to which targets can expose you. How often do you think people sacrifice their goals and achieve their goals? The average is only once. Most of them give up before they even try. And why give up all barriers, challenges such issues that soon emerge when they choose to do something they've never done before. Nonetheless, successful people are much more failing than the others. Successful people encounter more, break, recompose

117

and seek again and again until they are finally victorious. Those who struggle to excel learned a few things, but soon resigned themselves to returning to what they did before. Resolve, never lose. Pursue your ambitions vigorously. Go through your life and recognize the possibilities for your decision to continue to be the key to success. Whenever you have any trouble or discouragement, consider these observations. Think also about what you can do to solve your problems and reach your goals now and start straight away! Never give up. Never give up.

Learn the Power of Becoming a True Stoic Male

A few things are in our control, and others aren't. Things that we control are our thoughts, interests, what we want, abhorrence's, and, in a word, whatever are our actions. Things not in our control are body, property, notoriety, direction, and, in a single word, whatever are not our actions

You are born on this beautiful, strange planet which is as it should be. Your family, relatives, mother, and father celebrated the introduction of a person in this world. A youngster is developed by sustenance, support from his folks - the mother, adores him, gives her life to him, the father's employment, in any case, is a remarkable one, which we have to turn into. Dauntless, the gallant, discipline his child, so that, he can figure out how to master the genuine manly power. There are situations, where the tyke loses his father, because of unexpected yet avoidable/unavoidable conditions, which transforms the youthful tyke into defiant, presumptuous grown-up! This section is for that blackguard who lost his father or for the person who anticipates that his father should comprehend the complexities of human connections and live for once a solid male!

Who is a Stoic? Also, how to turn into the True Male.

"Stoic" is a word to portray a person, who shows fewer feelings, or who talks less. Stoicism was a Philosophy established by Zino of Citium in Greece. It was polished, as a way of life was Epictetus - who was born as a slave in Hierapolis, Phrygia, present-day Turkey. Epictetus figured out how to apply the Stoic standards, and never was defeated from the difficulties tossed at him. His master, at one moment, wounded his leg, but then, he grinned and told his master in a calm tone; "See, I disclosed to you, my leg would break." Through Epictetus, we can create and develop the propensity for turning into a True Stoic Male.

Presently, as we start examining, and slashing the practices on turning into a Stoic male, we should inspect now somewhat profoundly on who this person is. Regardless of whether you'd like this new change in your character, personality, your folks, companions, relatives, may see you as egotistical. However, you will be loaded up with calmness, tranquillity calling every one of the Gods, gathering to you the power to master any situation, condition and just controlling your considerations and actions. Presently, that is a power you should learn and follow. The following are a couple of pills taken from Epictetus' lessons. You should bite and swallow regular! These pills are not delectable, yet they are here to give you the total power inside yourself, and not depend on others for your weakness, situations which you see are crazy.

Let Death and outcast, and every single other thing which seems horrendous be day by day before your eyes, yet necessarily Death and you will win and never engage any miserable idea, nor too anxiously want anything.

Life is a battle. You can't escape now, Death is the only way. Terrifying yet, this is the last answer before leaving Earth. We are in pursuit of our wants - money, vocation, ladies, desire, power, an extraordinary house, connections. All these outer things are neither terrible nor useful for a Stoic. All these appear to be indifferent to a Stoic. If somebody discovers a person who lost his money, was dismissed by a lady and is as calm as water, he will begin to ask - why this person is so cold, or refreshing, untethered from this reality. If a situation ever appears to be crazy, envision how God Zeus might take control of the situation. That is the thing that Epictetus said to his understudies while he was encouraging Stoicism back in Rome.

Token Mori (recall, one day you also beyond words)

There is no real way to put this yet recollect; your time is running out! In this way, what should a Stoic Male accomplish that guarantees him not to append anything outside and have full oversight over himself? Get yourself a Goal! You need a mission present to challenge yourself. Hit the Gym today, and fabricate your build, lift weights, and eat that torment, since Stoic is indifferent to agony and joy. Need to construct another skill? Practice every day like you loathe doing, meet individuals, get familiar with their shrouded expectations, read their small scale inconspicuous feelings, figure out how to be calm like a stone, talk less, let your actions do the talking. Your time is constrained, so realize where to invest your energy - Decoding individuals, mastering a new skill, or attempting to assemble your definitive structure.

Be generally quiet, or talk only about what is essential, and in fewer words.

Guarantee not to permit your giggling to be excessive; on numerous events, nor bountiful like a lunatic. Indeed, this is extremely difficult. We, as a whole, prefer to split on - cruel jokes, and this can help the state of mind. What's more, this is one power you can use in your life. A state in which your manager puts you down or your dear companion sold out despite your good faith or your cherished one spits at you. You can use your Amused Mastery, as though, you discovered what sort of person he/she was. Concur and Amplifying to situations, for example, considering you a Bastard, pointless, and reframing to your world gives you another power wherein you can rehearse.

If a person gave your body to someone more peculiar, he met on his way, you would unquestionably be irate. Also, do you feel no disgrace in giving over your very own brain to be confounded and mystified by any individual who happens to ambush you verbally?

At long last your quietness, your words amount to nothing if you couldn't close a bonehead with your word. A genuine Stoic like Cato, utilizes his words sparingly, why, since you lose any fight if you have to demonstrate your value. Cato's Action did the talking. He was prepared to execute himself to oust Julius Caesar from the position of authority (which he in the long run achieved)

We are working up a resilient person who lost his expectations, dreams from the truth, learning while at the same time teaching ourselves to grasp the power of manliness swimming through your veins and feel an absolute control living inside you. Keep in mind this: What stays in this world is your inheritance. The amount of value you are as a person. If you need to test an absolute power between human interactions, begin perusing the 48 laws of power. Those are a portion of the genuine thick pills to swallow!

Chapter 7: Confidence Boosters

Positive self-esteem

Positive self-esteem refers to a general similarity between you and others. You are more confident about yourself, you believe in your own abilities, and you can be a happier, more successful person. Once you know about confidence boosters and how they increase self-esteem, it's a simple job to apply them to your life. Taking care of yourself physically and mentally increases endurance and helps you to cope with challenges every day. Doing fun things helps you to lead a happier life. The people you associate with and build relationships with have a drastic impact on your own worth. Are you friends the people who keep putting you down, or are they the kind of people who praise you if you are successful? You have to stick around people who want you to be content to have high self-esteem and be satisfied.

Protective self-esteem

people with protective self-esteem have positive opinions about themselves but are vulnerable to criticism and delicate. When questioned by an official, they would blame or apologize others rather than recognize their responsibility. We don't know how to answer in a non-defensive way unlike people with positive self-esteem. These types of people constantly need to be strengthened in order to increase their trust. I always feel the need to bring others down to feel good.

Low self-esteem

Low self-esteem is something many young people are dealing with. It can be a result of numerous factors, such as genetics, physical appearance, violence, abuse and social status. Those who have low self-esteem are unable to integrate confidence boosters in their lives if their peers have positive self-esteem. When suggestions or compliments are given, they frequently take it personally and become self-critical and nervous. We often have unsatisfactory relationships and are unable to achieve our goals. Depression is also a low self-esteem trait. In some cases, it even gets so high that they don't know how to deal with life anymore; they tend to hurt themselves and often contemplate suicide in some cases.

Self-confidence is a part of all of us. It is a product of our experiences, our ties, our goals and our actions. Although living with low self-esteem can seem like a daunting, relentless struggle, it can improve. The first move is to think about confidence boosters. The real task is to apply them. This sticks with you and influences the course of your life until you change your mindset and attitude.

Learn How to Alter Your Life With to Self Esteem

Here's a fundamental fact that I think you already know:' good self-esteem is the key to success.' Regardless of whether it is friendships, jobs, social life, economy, you're still going to need good self-esteem. So how can we develop self-appreciation?

Let's look at it as an issue. 1–defining the problem, 2 – considering it, 3–seeing the solutions,4–implementing a solution. Simple! Easy! (I know it's not that easy, but let's do it.) 1. Defining the issue–generally, self-esteem means contrasting oneself to others. We all classify people, respect and look at some people, neglect or talk to others, deliberately or subconsciously, (horrible but real), everything is how we feel about ourselves about other people-we give ourselves a mental sign of our position in society. You think that we are worthless, everyone's better than us, and we're never going to get anywhere, you think, what's that point?'

It is because you have a misunderstanding about yourself, and this is the heart of the problem. Why is this a misconception? You are too self-critical because you have put the poor quality on yourself when contrasting yourself with others.

2. Think of it—let's use a metaphor first. Low self-esteem is like you have put something in a shop window with a wrong price card. Let's say that the items in the shop were you and your colleagues at work. You are all doing the same thing, you are all being compensated in the same ways, but the shop manager has placed $100 price tag on them and $1 on you, you're all doing the same thing because he clearly made a mistake..... and imagine who is the boss responsible for putting the wrong price ticket in a store-you're the one who handles your life. You can, therefore, correct this by increasing the price, i.e., by raising and creating your love for yourself.

Second, self-esteem is not something in your blood; you often see brothers and sisters, which have very contrasting personalities. The good news is that it can be learned how to build up or gain self-esteem. Interesting fact, did you know that around 60 per cent of us have low self-esteem according to surveys? You certainly aren't alone, though. It, I believe, is because we are not encouraged to deal with life, criticize and reverse, etc. from an early age or in the school a non-criticism seems to me-everybody succeeds mindset, but it does not teach you how to build up your self-esteem.

3. Look at the remedies-You need some self-analysis to get a real objective view of yourself to see how to develop self-esteem. We all have strengths and weaknesses, write them down, once we understand them, we can build on them. What are you best at? What are you bad at? What do you like? What do you like to do? What do you want to be reasonable about? What are you doing wrong? What do you not like to do?

Next, describe what you care about. Don't think your boss or the opposite sex's congratulations are very significant, it can feel good, but it won't last. Concentrate on bigger things. We want to know and surpass our potential and achieve things-think in this direction.

Now everybody is different, but you must understand that you will need to improve to develop your self-esteem. There will be nothing more if you don't. Here's a broad list, look at it, if you want to add, select the right ones, be frank, look at the strengths and weaknesses of yourself, and see how they relate.

Self-respect-stop beating yourself, eradicate any criticism of yourself.

Attitude–bad things happen, be optimistic, concentrate not on the issue but on the solution. Treat failure as a lesson and not as a reversal.

Relationships-mixes of positive people rather than negative ones.

Human knowledge-Take patience, compassion, polity, and good manners. Respect and listen to and understand other people's needs.

Take a look at your social customs.

Switch embrace-don't be afraid or cynical.

Share, work, and connect 4. 4. Focus on improving the above abilities, focus on them. Beset in perspective–this is the most important thing.

Visualize your career success, socially or in relationships, but have the right values. Visualization is a powerful tool often used by sports professionals and helps you develop self-esteem.

You will consider when you learn how to build your self-esteem, to be more effective in working, socially, and in relationships. It's like a downward spiral, which leads to unhappiness and hinders you from doing anything–don't give up, be determined.

Building of Teen Self Esteem Starts at Birth

When does self-appreciation start? We often believe that self-esteem in our children starts when they reach their two years, not realizing that it starts at birth. It is developed from the very beginning with the influence of parental attitudes and behaviours and then continues into all development in children.

First of all, they build their self-esteem by meeting their basic needs, including the need for love, comfort, and closeness. How their parents or caregivers treat children sets the stage for the development of self-esteem. Young babies and children who feel unloved find it harder to develop a sense of self-worth and then take them into later childhood and into their adolescence.

Supporting parental behaviour, including encouraging and praising accomplishments and internalizing the parent's attitudes toward success and failure, are the most critical factors in early childhood self-esteem. Stress in your home, like parents arguing a lot or having friends with whom to play and interact, can negatively impact the self-esteem and self-worth of a child at a very young age.

When kids have high self-esteem, they can deal with conflict, pressure from peers, and make friends easier. In this stage, children learn self-confidence by developing their senses of confidence, independence, and initiative with parents and siblings and then interacting with friends and relatives.

Self-esteem comes from various sources for children at different developmental stages. During our youth, our self-esteem is instilled in us. It is essential to be aware whether the current situation in the home is critical; since parents and family members blame themselves tend to rob the child of their feelings of self-worth gradually.

Self-esteem is defined as being inwardly pleasant. This is how you perceive yourself and your self-worth. When it reflects within your child, it is what you think and feels about yourself and how well you think that you do things, it is ultimately essential, and it is on this basis that your self-esteem builds.

As kids grow up and mature and their observations move within their homes and into school, and with their peers, how they determine their self-esteem becomes more critical in these areas. Schools also have an enormous impact on self-esteem by fostering competitive attitudes and diversity and recognizing academic, sports, and arts achievements. Social acceptance by a peer group of children is essential at this stage in developing and maintaining self-esteem.

The emotional and physical change in adolescence, especially in early teens, presents a child's self-esteem with new challenges. The time when teens undergo significant changes in life, self-esteem may be very fragile, they face physical and hormonal changes. This is the moment when young people want and need a supportive family.

Adjusting in your environment is increasingly important to your self-esteem, and relationships with the opposite or sometimes same gender, in later adolescence, can become a significant source of confidence or insecurity. Body image is a critical element of teenagers ' self-esteem, and how their peers see them is of great concern. For both boys and girls, body images are essential, and teens who like their look and accept themselves the way they are, have high self-confidence.

Parents can encourage self-esteem by expressing their affection and support for the child and help the child to start as previously stated in the early years, rather than imposing unreachably high standards, set realistic goals for achievement. Young people who learn to set goals in their lives have higher self-esteem than people who do not. In this time and even before, visualization can be taught to children and adolescents. This is an excellent tool to create and develop self-esteem for all people, and visualization videos are a great tool.

Teens could also be encouraged to watch the words they use to describe themselves, for example, if they always say they're stupid, or that they can't succeed, then, make it a habit of saying positive things and use this positive attitude to give you full self-esteem. The use of affirmations is also an excellent way, to begin with, the affirmation language, which can also be used in vision map videos.

Make sure and tell your teen that nobody is flawless in the eyes of everyone else, so you can only brace yourself for disappointment and failure by striving to become perfect. Spend more time focusing on the things you appreciate and less on those you don't like. Teach them to trust themselves fully, and others will also trust and believe in them.

Chapter 8: Lower Self-Esteem and Cause of Depression

We have a higher risk of depression if our self-esteem is small, which is characteristic of codependency. Maladaptive behaviour is acquired, and the values and self-esteem and habits that cause low self-esteem and codependency are therefore learned. Self-esteem is what we feel of ourselves. We think of ourselves. Positive and negative self-assessments are included. Good self-esteem is a real, optimistic perception of oneself. This represents respect for oneself and implies a sense of value, which is not defined by contrast with others or approval. Self-acceptance (included by some writers in mutual-esteem) is even more profound. It feels good enough, not ideal, not incomplete. They believe that we are worth and loved, not just due to appearance, talent, accomplishment, intellect, rank, or popularity. It's a feeling of deep fulfilment.

All of us have intrinsic value, not dependent on our success or what we do or offer. Just as every baby and race is exceptional and caring, so are we. Regrettably, many of us as codependents grew up in families with no affection, conditional love, or won. We figured we had to gain or win a parent's attention. As a consequence, we hate being honest because of fear that we may be unhappy. We must follow people who can't love or deny lovers. In interactions and at work, we "over-do" and "over-give," and finally feel resentful, manipulated, or abused.

If you think that self-esteem is important for living and having healthy relationships, enjoying and enduring, you are wrong! The following bad habits, common to codependents, can make you feel insecure, embarrassed, depressed, sad, and hopeless:

- Negative comparing yourself with others.

- You may find fault with yourself

- tyrannizing yourself in "Should."

- Project self-criticism with others and believe they judge you.

- Feeling "better than" is a sure way to offset the underlying guilt and

- low self-confidence.

- The lift we're getting is wrong. It would be better to ask why we have to equate ourselves to someone else.

- It's self-shaming when we compare ourselves negatively.

- We feel lower, we lose trust, and we like less.

- It depresses and discourages our mood.

An active "inner critic" assassinates us with what we ought to and ought not to do and assaults what we have already done. Usual discovery of faults can lead us to believe that others see us as we see ourselves. This way, we project our criticism towards others and expect and feel the effect of criticism or judgment, even if no objection exists.

Reduced self-confidence makes us afraid to make mistakes, to look stupid, or to fail. Our self-esteem is always on the line, and it is, therefore, safer to try nothing new to avoid incompetence or failure. This is another reason why we continue to create unique and strenuous activities or experiences. At the same time, we criticize ourselves for not achieving our objectives. Instead of taking a chance, we are wrong not to try, which means "failure" and low self-esteem.

Adjusting others from a young age leaves us uncertain about our values and beliefs and promotes trust in others. It becomes challenging to make choices, even paralyzing. Low self-esteem and guilt raise our concern that mistakes lead to self-doubt, weakness, and indecision. Slightly, we procrastinate and look for affirmation, feedback, and reactions that further weaken our self-confidence and self-esteem.

Adapting to others also alienates us from our needs and desires. They tell ourselves and others that they are not essential by not understanding, communicating, and satisfying our needs and wants. On the other hand, it creates self-esteem by taking responsibility to meet our needs and demanding (such as requesting an increase). If not, we feel helpless, a victim of circumstances, and others.

The respect and love that we deny ourselves makes us vulnerable to abuse and exploitation. We do not feel worthy of well being handled and refuse to be humiliated or disregarded, justify, or rationalize. Based on the acceptance of others, we are wary of setting limits so that we do not alienate those we love or need. We quickly blame ourselves and accept blame from others because we're guilty of shame. Although we forgive others ' mistakes, mainly when we are excused, we are not as kind to ourselves. Excuses for us don't count. In reality, due to past mistakes, we can punish ourselves and blame ourselves for years.

Treatment for low self-esteem and depression Hopefully,

we will increase our self-esteem and our self-fulfilment potential. This enhances our imagination, goals, physical and emotional wellbeing, affection, and resilience in the face of adversity. It is essential for performance.

How Low Self Esteem Affects Our Wellbeing

Self Esteem is defined as a psychological state based on an individual's assessment of its importance. The definition describes a person's point of view as to whether or not they are worthy of praise. Briefly, your self-esteem defines the metric you want.

Low Self Estima is a word that we use to describe people who don't think very much about themselves. People with low self-esteem have a little self-worth measure. You don't feel good about who and what you are. This can create any number of problems for the person experiencing the condition.

Low self-esteem also may be defined simply as "feeling insecure." Low self-esteem can include the following common indicators: relying too heavily on others for decisions and guidance and frequently feeling overwhelmed by normal life pressures, feeling more depressed than others physically: appearance, age, height, weight, etc. Such patterns are superficial, and we appear to associate them automatically with more optimistic or over-trustful personalities. Besides, these measures reflect a kind of over-compensation designed to hide feelings of failure or inferiority. These might include the following: general frustration and a need for Quick vengeance fuse, prone to regular irritations that quickly escalate to outbursts. Conflictive, immediately confronted, and violently reply Blaming issue with others. Argumentation over trivial or insignificant issues. Although it is a common condition, and we are all familiar with it, many would identify it as a disorder or disease. This has been addressed, but low self-esteem fulfils many requirements describing conditions. For example, low self-esteem can be uncontrollable; for many, it shows similar symptoms and seems to be related to similar past experiences such as violence in many situations. People with low self-esteem may be more vulnerable to other health problems because of the added pressures which this disorder frequently accompanies.

Something good is that we can boost our self-esteem through rigorous training and disciplined practice. As we regain our self-esteem, we begin to move back into prosperous and more successful, enjoyable lives. We can do many things every day to improve our self-esteem. There are some things to do next.

Avoid being attacked. Punishing yourself for perceived failures only over time can decrease your self-esteem.

Work to achieve your goals. Each day, strive to advance to at least one of the goals of your life. Be patient and devote yourself to doing so every day. It strengthens your confidence and takes you closer to your dreams.

Please fill your mind with positive data. Read books on self-help. Participate in trust courses. Research and return to the things that inspire you.

Make an effort. Make efforts. Do try to accomplish assignments and challenges. When you excel, it will strengthen your self-esteem and confidence. It won't matter if you fail, because you know you've done your hardest.

Emphasize your strengths and note them as often as possible. Use them to deal with difficult circumstances.

Identify areas of difficulty and bad habits. If you're frustrated, learn to identify it and stop until it gets out of hand. It takes practice to change bad habits but immediate positive results. Think of all the negative situations you can prevent by not negatively affecting the climate.

Visualize every day, your performance. When you wake up, imagine yourself fulfilling your goals and becoming the person you want to be. This is your inspiration to make an honest effort every day to come closer to this potential reality.

Affirmations. Comments. Mind your positive characteristics as often as you can. Speak openly to them. Be brave. Be bold.

Concentrate on growth. Never look back. The past has nothing to do with it. Seek and follow your wishes every day.

Know how you can quit by taking yourself seriously. Everything doesn't have to be so awful sometimes. Relax, and have fun. Learn to be humble and smile at yourself. We're all wrong. We're humorous sometimes.

Be yourself. You can do whatever you want, but you can't be somebody else. Learn to accept all your faults and yourself. You can improve them, and you can refine them. You don't describe your shortcomings.

When you find that you need to boost your self-esteem, hold specific suggestions close at hand. Self-esteem is a vital part of life. This influences our emotions, our way of functioning, and our way of interacting with the world around us. If you acquire low self-esteem, it can affect anything you think about and make you feel negative. It can influence all you do in all aspects of your life. Going through life with low self-esteem is like swimming with the attached links.

Free yourself from low self-respect, and your life will be better in innumerable ways.

The Mystery Surrounding Self-Esteem

Every person creates self-esteem in whatever fields he is commanding.

If you kill love, you kill the person.

Low self-esteem denies an individual the opportunity to be themselves. Psychologists mostly work with the person affected trying to mend their damaged trust, but no one tells us that there is more to the cycle of managing this mess than just the people changed.

Low self-esteem frustrates a human being and can lead to depression or even worse, suicide. Unfortunately, it is not well understood, and more of a personal problem is considered during the development phases. It only becomes a family problem if it has been discouraged.

Without everyone taking personal responsibility for this rapidly growing "low self-esteem" family, devastation can get out of hand more than it does, right from home to other institutions.

Who is responsible for low self-esteem?

Looking at yourself, you can feel so confident that you have never contributed to lowering the confidence of someone else! As long as you relate to people every day, you may be part of somebody else's appreciation.

Your closest family members are most concerned since you feel the pain if you lose. Nonetheless, note that what affects your child may be an example of what you did to an alien.

Some acts that reduce self-esteem. As teachers, if you humiliate a poor student at any point, you can trigger a withdrawal syndrome in him and affect him after that. You don't think an adolescent knows how his teacher mocked him for poor performance. And worse, he knows the name of the instructor. You might not be able to persuade him if he is an average student that he can do better.

The analogy is an admired killer. People take responsibility for a pending occurrence at a conference. Somebody favours one task to another, then suddenly, someone yells, "kids can even perform better than you." The consequences of such a declaration may not be as clear as this assertion, depending on the makeup.

Constant complaints about the same person decrease his self-esteem — I don't like the style. You can't be serious about that simple thing, and you don't understand it. I didn't like your Bible study contribution.

You mean you can't drive faster?

The first questions that will arise before the victims are, "will it be an error?" Does low self-esteem affect every victim? "Am I about to ask a stupid question?"

You can smile and wonder why, given your bad experiences, you are not a patient with poor self-esteem.

The reason for this is simple. That individual is created uniquely. Sadly, we expect people to be like us most of the time, rather than recognizing that we can't be the same.

One vigorous man cleans his wounds instantly, while another one cries for three days for a similar injury. The later may have low self-esteem. It's not his fault, but he's just so wired.

What are the consequences of increasing the trust of the people?

In the long term, you will also suffer because if the individual does not become himself, you are part of the suffering. Suppose this is your child or wife; you can't escape.

In such a case, since he is in a mental state, he can not unleash his power. His overall growth is astounding. No matter how much he tries to lean on a shoulder when you are in need, he can not, with the same love.

Once it progresses to depression, you will spend unexpected sums of money to solve a problem you might have avoided.

Who causes lower self-esteem?

You know that, and others don't know.

Supposing the characters of people are close to yours, and they are not concerned about such humiliation.

Use your power to put the other down. A child is powerless regardless of age and may neglect what he or she does but still has low self-esteem.

How to avoid reducing people's appreciation. Begin by accepting that people should not be like you.

Consider the qualities you see in others instead of the flaws.

Correct errors in a friendly way, if possible.

Don't talk about someone else's weakness if you're not looking for a solution to it.

Never laugh at someone's face for an error.

Prepare to apologize only if your words have sent an inappropriate message.

Listen and answer only when he's quiet. Speak only when he finishes, let him feel like his intellect is being compromised and heightened.

How to let go of low self-esteem while it advances. Always listen to what makes no sense to you and engage. You're living with your loved ones, after all.

Create an environment that is pleasant and easily accessible.

How to deal with an adult who is suffering from low self-esteem. Answer his questions immediately. It makes him feel unwelcome by ignoring or dismissing him.

Get much closer than ever to him; your lack of concern is an emotional lure.

Give him a chance to make and execute decisions. Congratulations on all the efforts that have been created.

Encourage him to share real stories of people who have experienced similar events.

Gradually let him know that there may be a misunderstanding of the disparity between personalities where this was not supposed to be.

Can low self-appreciation last forever?

If you have to deal with it yourself, it may last forever or not. It depends on what the victim wants, or even knows first of all, and it's a question.

There are only two ways of doing this. Either you choose to get out of it or accept the situation as it is. You have to tackle the cause of the problem to make a difference. Let the individual know the effects in your life of his acts and prove that you can't live with them. If he hurts you, heighten the warning to alert you and do it politically.

The best of all educators is an experience. Sharing is a matter of concern.

The environment makes people what they are. Whatever the challenge you seek to be yourself, people willingly or unconsciously transform it into a generic image. If mature adults happen, you can imagine the effects on children or adolescents! This interferes with authentic self-esteem, which mostly decreases this.

Have you ever engaged in reducing self-esteem?

Have you handled a low self-esteem victim?

What have you been through?

Advice to anyone who wants to secure the trust of his child instead of trying to restore it?

Chapter 9: Permanently Ending Procrastination

Why does procrastination cause pressure?

Another regular yet unavoidable wellspring of worry in present-day society is procrastination, or continually putting off the finishing of tasks.

Procrastination is viewed as a stressor since it frequently causes deferrals and powers people to pack finally. Procrastination this way prompts many increasingly unpleasant circumstances.

Procrastination can take a few structures:

99% of the time, people experience lament after they have procrastinated because they have less time to finish what they ought to have begun some time prior.

A person may feel fulfilled and cheerful while procrastinating; however, it's a different story when due dates start to a shut-in, and the slacker understands that he had officially 'spent' a large portion of the available time that he has.

Why do people procrastinate?

To beat procrastination, we need to comprehend why people routinely resort to it in any case:

Performing more straightforward tasks for beginning the more difficult ones.

Picking pleasurable exercises over progressively essential exercises.

Playing out a progression of less essential exercises so you won't need to begin one.

1. **Discomfort** - it is a well-known fact that each significant undertaking or activity includes some degree of pain. Applying exertion and spending vitality on something is essential to create substantial results.

When a person has a shallow threshold for mental, enthusiastic, or physical discomfort, he may procrastinate to postpone encountering discomfort.

A low threshold is the most widely recognized purpose behind putting off different exercises. More often than not, people are unconscious of their discomfort thresholds; thus, the decision to procrastinate is driven by an intuitive want to stay away from discomfort.

2. **Fear of a Failing** - Some grown-ups are so scared of coming up short at something that they just put off getting things done for whatever length of time that they can.

When a person fears disappointment, they imagine all the mental and enthusiastic discomforts that they will understand if they don't prevail with regards to achieving a task attractively. People who put stock in compulsiveness are bound to procrastinate because of a general fear of disappointment.

3. **Fear of Rejection** - There are a few circumstances where a completely fit grown-up ends up reluctant to accomplish something since he feels that somebody

(almost like a specialist figure) will object to their activities.

This fear is established in the conviction that other people's valuations are substantially more significant than your self-valuation. For instance, a person who has needed to figure out how to paint may procrastinate inconclusively because they feel that other people will say that their works of art are standard or terrible.

4. **Refusal to Do Something** - When a person feels that it is uncalled for that they need to accomplish something, they will generally abstain from doing the said task for whatever length of time that conceivable.

A person may turn out to be progressively baffled and furious as the due date for the task draws near. When they need to work twice or three times as hard to complete the job, the person can turn out to be considerably progressively worried about this circumstance.

1. **Don't Overthink** - Overthinking something is never a decent decision since it is debilitating to cycle similar

considerations in a single's psyche more than once, while never depending on activity.

Rather than considering accomplishing something over and over, do what needs to be done. Keep in mind Nike's motto, "get it done?" It's the ideal trademark for staying away from procrastination!

2. **Change Your Mindset** - Many people procrastinate because they need to defer discomfort or strain.

Rather than imagining that you are liberating yourself of any discomfort, consider procrastination drawing out the trouble since you'll wind up recollecting every one of the things you need to do, regardless of whether you're not doing them right now.

3. **Plan Ahead -** If you feel restless about the result of something you need to do, you can lessen your nervousness or questions by making a plan ahead of time. Make sure to record the subtleties of what you need to do and your whole project.

Ordinarily, we see things differently when they're determined to paper. Items that have all the earmarks of being awful or too testing seem more straightforward to control and oversee when you record the precise subtleties if this works for you at that point, rehash this procedure whenever you feel like procrastinating.

If at least one of the reasons expressed above concerns you, realize that these are on the whole merely mental states and you can deliberately supersede them for increasingly positive and profitable conduct.

Self-Hypnosis Benefits and Limitations

Much has been said about self-hypnosis lately. Let us think about what self-hypnosis is before we get to what it can and can not do for us. If you've ever been with hypnotherapists, they might have told you that all Hypnosis is self-hypnosis. This is true. What this means is that without your consent or participation, no one can make you hypnotic. The news and the stage hypnotizers have led many to believe that Hypnosis is not a natural state that those with mental control could place on us.

Nothing could go beyond the facts. Hypnosis is a natural state of mind in which we all join multiple times a day. If your attention is so concentrated that you don't know what's happening around you, you're in a hypnotic state. While watching TV or reading or playing, we are in a state of Hypnosis once we get out of the present and into our minds and focus our attention.

There are other times when we are in a hypnotic light state. We are in a highly suggestible state, for example, when called into the office. We're in light Hypnosis when we are in a large crowd at a concert or another event. These are just a few examples when, in our regular daily lives, we are in Hypnosis.

From these examples, we can understand that Hypnosis is a state of the mind in which we concentrate on something other than what is happening right before us, or that we focus so much on what is in front of us that we lose consciousness of everything else. It is a condition in which we are suggestible so that we can internalize and integrate knowledge into our fact or belief system. An example is when we watch a film and eventually cry. Though the events have not happened to us, we are so committed that we feel the feelings they feel.

When we think therapeutically about self-hypnosis, we don't talk about these experiences. We speak about a systematic process by taking our attention away from our current environment and place ourselves in an altered state of mind for a particular purpose.

So how are we going to make self-hypnosis?

There are so many ways to make self-hypnosis, but I will explain a simple yet effective method for this writing that everyone can do.

The first thing you want to do is to find a quiet place to stay. Grant yourself half an hour. Give yourself a quarter. Turn off your phone and tell the children to remain calm and have fun at this time. Nonetheless, in an emergency, realize that you can quickly awaken and return to ordinary waking consciousness.

Get relaxed, sit, or lie down. If you like, you can have soft music in the background. Most meditative music recordings are suitable for self-hypnosis. Many may use music to relax more profoundly.

Concentrate on your breathing now. Watch your breath come and go out of your nose. Feel the wind reaching your body. Look at your belly rising and falling. A breathing exercise is often followed by thinking "Respire in calmness and relaxation, and respire stress and tension." You can also use meditation to bring you down to a deep calmness. Imagine your eyes ' muscles start to relax and slump. And take the sensation to the top of your head. Feel the full relaxation of all the muscles in your chest, face, and neck. Use this method to go through the entire body, calmly and soothingly.

Use terms in your mind such as "deeper and deeper into relaxation," "walking down," "quiet relaxed relaxation," etc. as the stress is going out of your muscles and breathing.

Returning is another excellent way to get further into relaxation. "10 going down, nine times as relaxed as before, eight still going down... and so on," you may feel a physical feeling like floating, tingling, or numbness. You may feel a temperature change, whether warming or refreshing. Everyone has a different hypnosis experience. Beware of your senses and see how you are going to experience Hypnosis.

Most people will ask at this level, "What is the difference between self-hypnosis and meditation?" Meditation is a way of clearing the mind. Hypnosis is similar because you can relax and track your pulse, but the similarities end here. Hypnosis has a specific intention, and the mind is especially active, rather than becoming transparent, although in a different way from your normal state of consciousness.

You will be intentionally hypnotized. For example, if you use Hypnosis to relieve stress, you might want to' be calm and relaxed throughout your day. You may do this several times or envision and imagine the pressure that exists in your body through your fingers and toes. It may look like static electricity, or you may see angry gnomes marching out of the ends of your feet. Imagination plays an essential part in Hypnosis. It allows you to perceive and imagine the outcome you need. Two, feel refreshed, restful and energetic... three, feeling in the space your body... four, recalling every good thing you said today in my subconscious mind... five, open your eyes up. "Relax and take a few moments to return to your normal tolerance. Remember, when you give yourself an idea to repeat a few times, it takes you to get your mind in the first place. It's called compounding, the more you say it, the easier it is."The question is good. Here's a reply: the title of this chapter is' Self-hypnosis advantages and restrictions.' The term hypnotic and the hypnotherapist have a significant difference, the first being the state of mind, and the second being the treatment. You can bring so much wellness with self-hypnosis.

Now I can hear you asking, "Why would I go to a hypnotherapeutic if I could do it all on my own?" The response is: "Self-hypnosis advantages and drawbacks" is the heading of this post. There is a significant difference between the terms hypnosis and hypnotherapist. One is a mental condition and one in counselling.

Through self-hypnosis, you can do a lot of good. If you want, you can reduce blood pressure. You may relieve pressure and enhance sleep patterns. You can strengthen your models of learning. Most things can be done with self-hypnosis. Yet one essential thing that you can't do with self-hypnosis is therapy.

The distinction between a hypnotherapist and hypnotherapy is the care. A hypnotherapist uses psychological techniques while the client is hypnotized to make life changes. Hypnotherapy is a relationship between the hypnotherapist and the patient. Someone who has Hypnosis can not ask questions or dig deeper and use the necessary tools to discover the source of an issue or to communicate with their inner child therapeutically. For these results, a hypnotherapist needs to work with it.

Self-hypnosis is very useful in reducing stress and other related problems. It's essential to have a hypnotherapist work with you to get to the heart of a problem and to find solutions for a healing experience.

If you are looking for a hypnotherapist, find someone you are confident with. Make sure they're qualified to do the job. Check your credentials, if possible. No government agency controls hypnotherapy so that someone can hang a shingle and call himself a hypnotherapist. Ensure that the person with whom you deal with is well educated and skilled in their business practice. It's better to take your time before choosing the right hypnotherapist than to find out that you made a mistake later.

Start your body-hypnosis and feel what it is and what it can do for you, and then go and see the right psychotherapist for you.

Declutter Ideas You Can Use

Are you looking for inspiration to declutter?

Perhaps it's your life or your home that you need to declutter. However, you can't propel yourself to begin or complete the decluttering. This chapter will talk about specific ways that can give you the inspiration to declutter.

Most importantly, train yourself to get the correct outlook. Continue advising yourself that unorganized people make straightforward employments hard for themselves. Chaotic people frequently do a similar activity again and again, and continuously burn through valuable time searching for things. People who are organized, and have decluttered their homes well, and can keep over it are in harmony with themselves and are happy with their lives.

Another approach to persuade yourself to dispose of clutter is by spending time with companions who live in clutter-free homes. Visit them frequently at their homes and propel yourself by their instances of decluttering, approach your companions for exhorting and their insider facts to declutter free homes. Perhaps you could even request that they help you with decluttering your home. You could likewise join a decluttering gathering on the internet, where numerous people join to spur each other to move toward becoming clutter-free.

You could likewise rouse yourself to declutter, by marking the calendar for a special event; like hosting a birthday get-together at home, or welcoming companions or somebody special around your home for supper. Be reasonable and give yourself a lot of time to manage the clutter. Make an arrangement and stick to it. Doubtlessly you will need to have a beautiful, clean home to be glad for when your companions or that special somebody comes around for supper, that should give you enough inspiration to declutter.

You may have some declutter ideas and may even utilize them yet at the same time; you feel that there are increasingly imaginative approaches to deal with clutter. A lot of writes-up and books will give you steps on when, how, and where to begin with the undertaking.

There is nothing more humiliating than having unforeseen visitors when your home is cluttered with such a large number of things. You can make sure that this will harm you. It is always a decent practice to declutter when you can make just as perfect and organized home.

You may not be the individual who likes to do research and find out about strategies on the most proficient method to declutter. A large portion of your ideas originates as a matter of fact and perception. You think about the organizational tools that you have to declutter like the checked boxes and the garbage bags. You know about decluttering each room or zone in turn. You have set declutter day plans just as the time to do it.

The majority of the mentioned above, you have done and keep on doing, yet there is one component that is effectively overlooked when it comes to decluttering. The fundamental key to having a sans clutter home is understanding why clutter occurs in the first place. You have to recognize that specific practices, whether yours or different members of the family unit is in charge of structured up clutter. So a significant declutter thought is to change frames of mind and conduct with positive abilities to have an organized life and condition.

When you have an organized home, there are a more significant number of advantages than having the place strewn with paper, toys, books, things, and so on. Without a doubt, feelings of anxiety increment, there will come a time when you can never again endure the clutter that you need to take care of.

The following are some declutter ideas that you can do directly after perusing this chapter . You can begin decluttering rooms and organize your life:

1. If you have constrained time in the first part of the day and you need to make pack lunch for you or the kids, place all that you need in one territory the previous night. This will make planning time quicker.

2. Have the children set up their school things? Give them a chance to place books and different materials inside their bags the previous night.

3. Make it a standard to place handbag, keys, portfolios, bags, and so on in an assigned region, so you generally realize where to discover them and maintain a strategic distance from the clutter.

4. Abstain from having dirtied garments everywhere. Have clothing bins or hampers for filthy garments and those requiring cleaning. Place them close to the bathroom, entryways for family members to see.

5. Use shoe racks to organize footwear. Use tie racks for ties and scarves. Introduce snares for tops, caps, and handbags behind cabinet entryways. These organizational tools will give the cabinet an uncluttered look.

6. Place a net bag in the youngsters' rooms and let them place their stuffed toys and light material toys in

the net bag. This will show the kid right off the bat in life to return things to its appropriate place as to keep the room slick looking.

7. Make sure that each thing in your home has a place and that everybody knows where it is. Try not to place kitchen tools in the sanctum or your room. Family members should restore these things where they got the thing.

8. Have waste jars in each room and make it an approach to toss things in them appropriately. Make sure to let room proprietors take out their garbage every day and not permit any waste when they leave for school or the office.

9. A little crate is perfect for placing remote controls and other electronic contraption for the TV or stereo segment.

10. Examine with your family members that before bedtime, for in any event 15 minutes, they ought to declutter their rooms. Place everything all together. Give this a chance to be a propensity that youngsters can create.

The above are only some declutter ideas that will make home life better and organized. There are different sources online just as books that give top to bottom ideas for your reference.

Chapter 10: Benefits of a Decluttered Mind

Advantages of a Decluttered Mind

The best spot to start to declutter your life is from within. Numerous individuals neglect the advantages of a sound mind can offer. The mind can move towards becoming hindered with psychological weight and indeed sway an individual's capacity to work. Necessary leadership can turn into a test and adapting to issues may feel unthinkable when you don't have a clear mental state; in this manner, it is imperative to figure out how to free your mind of excessive clutter. Since everybody is different there is nobody size-fits-all strategy to clear your mind of clutter; nonetheless, coming up next are some basic methods that can start you on your adventure to decluttering your life by first decluttering your mind!

All in Good Time: Schedules

Lighten a portion of your mental stress by making a timetable. When you have all assignments sorted out and arranged out, with spare time included between, a significant measure of strain will be lifted. You will live more proficiently and suffer from less overpowering minutes. You can't get ready for everything, and calendars must be changed now and again. In any case, having a reliable schedule for the things you realize you should do, organized by significance, can have a considerable effect on your mental stress. Besides, this is an incredible method for promising you to have time put aside to rehearse your mind-decluttering systems.

Meditation for a Clear Mind

Meditation is a famous instrument to help declutter your life and your mind. You don't need to think as it was done in the good 'old days. Attempt this increasingly modernized system: start with music you appreciate. A few people profit by uplifting tunes or great songs, while others may prefer something edgier. The class is altogether up to you, and it doesn't need to be unwinding music. Next, locate a single region that you can disengage yourself from others and diversions.

Start by playing music. It is useful to have a playlist, or you can circle a similar song if you prefer, as long as you don't need to get up and restart the music when the song closes. The music is going about as a manual for the assistance you start to declutter your life. Get settled on a bed, love seat, seat or the floor. If you rest, ensure you don't nod off! Tune in to the music as it fills the zone around you. Close your eyes. Enable your body to unwind. It is ideal for lying on your back or sitting with your arms limp to advance total unwinding. Choose an essential sound in the song and tail it. Give your mind a chance to move towards becoming immersed in it as you trail the sound through the song. This enables your mind and body to concentrate on something different while unwinding and getting a charge out of good music.

Use Words to Remove Tension

Written words are an integral asset to declutter your life. How you utilize them is up to you. A few people prefer to write in a diary. This can be private, and nobody else needs to see it. If you are worried about others discovering your written musings, consider writing them down on a piece of paper and after that discarding it or demolishing it after you are finished.

Another suitable method to utilize written words is to compose letters. This is frequently done when pessimistic feelings emerge towards someone else in your life. When the message is written, store it someplace or discard it. The thought is to get your feelings out on the paper, instead of on the individual. This can work another route too. When you are feeling discouraged or down, pen a positive letter to a companion. This will help remind you of the good things so you can stay focused. You can even send the message if you need to! It is imperative to recall when you declutter your life, and you should endeavour to expel negative feelings and stay focused on the right things.

Start to declutter your life presently, beginning with your mind. You will feel better, work all the more adequately, and suffer from fewer misfortunes. Besides, when terrible things occur, you will be better prepared to deal with them when your mind is clear of clutter!

Dealing With Life And Over-Thinking

This should be the moment, after all the hard work, of the year, when we finally stop fretting and enjoy ourselves. But how do you prevent' what if' from nagging? Do you think about crowding back?

Sometimes we all do worry about things we have said or done, discuss deleted comments, or spend hours dissecting the significance of a specific e-mail or letter. We get pulled into a vortex of negative thoughts and emotions that rob our happiness and excitement almost without knowing it. It's a trend some psychologists call for. The initial thoughts lead to more negative thoughts and questions. The over-thought becomes a cascade that ferments and builds so that everything gets out of control. If you remain in this negative cycle, your life can be affected. It can also lead to some really bad decisions if relatively small issues become so fuzzy that you lose sight of them.

If we focus on what happened in the past (future), we actually destroy the moment we are in. You lack the here and now of your life to learn and appreciate.

Why are we doing this? The structure of our brain makes it easy to think over at the most basic level. Thoughts and memories are not only isolated and distinct from each other in our minds–they are linked together in complex networks of connections. One consequence of these deep interconnections is that thoughts about a certain issue in your life can trigger thoughts on other related questions.

Most of us have negative memories, potential worries, and doubts about the present. We're probably not aware of these negative thoughts most times. But if they come across us, even if it's because the climate is dreary or because we drink a lot of wine, it's easier to remember the negative memories and start the cycle of thought over. Most women are overwhelmed with household balancing responsibilities and feel the need to do all this perfectly. They tend to take responsibility for everyone, believe that we ought to be in charge and set ridiculously high expectations.

How can you tackle it? If you are a persistent thinker, you won't just be told to take time out and relax. You need to take active measures to control negative thinking and resolve it. Breaking the habit is not easy, and everyone has no magical solution, but these are some of the steps that experts say will help you break the negative cycle of thought.

1. Get a break-free mind from something to concentrate and boost your mood— whether it is reading a good book, walking the dog, getting a massage, or going to the fitness centre.

2. Take in hand–If you find the same thoughts going, ask yourself to stop firmly. Put yellow stickers as reminders on your desk and around the building.

3. Ditch the delaying tactics–If certain circumstances or locations cause thought, such as a desk filled with papers or unsolicited letters or e-mails, then do something about it, however low. Thinking that is related to inactivity could turn into a vicious cycle. Rather than living in fear of what you can't do and what

could happen, it's far easier to just deal with it by doing something.

4. Free your thoughts-questions that take on gigantic dimensions after frenetic concern can suddenly melt away when you speak to a friend. They could look ridiculous or funny. Finally, making a joke will help to alleviate your worries.

5. Time to think-decide when you can think. Time to think. Limit your time and stick to your timetable. Imagine holding all these thoughts in a special box at a particular time of the day, then seal them and turn them off at the end of the day.

6. Love the moment-plan things you enjoy actively. Anything that works for you doesn't matter what it is. It is hard to languish negatively when you have fun.

7. Express your emotions–Instead of constantly contemplating what your emotions actually mean, just

give yourself a switch. Weep, scream, kick a pillow, let your emotions feel, and proceed.

8. Forgive yourself–it doesn't mean to say that there have never been slight or negative remarks, but it doesn't mean to choose to put them aside instead of sitting on them.

9. Pay attention–Take time every day to be in the moment. It will not be quick, but it will continue, and you will reap the rewards. Watch the sunset in the backyard, spend 15 minutes in the park at lunchtime, and eat alone at a café. Don't banish your emotions, just let them go, but consider what's around you and how your body feels.

Countering Overthinking Towards an Improved Life

Let's just presume you hung around at a party, which was surrounded by friends and customers, and you meet someone you really want to talk to. Perhaps it's connected to a business, or you just want to establish personal ties. Whatever that is, you practice a mental twist of what you have to say as you do and plan to meet them, but you are left with a surprising fear at the back of your head. What if they don't want to talk to you? What if the dialogue line doesn't work? Or is it going awfully wrong? The uncertainty causes a kind of domino effect, and you start thinking of the worst thing that might be inevitable. With every thought, you are pulled deeper into the mystery twisted within your brain, which eventually prevents you from even speaking again. You then watch another person talk to the topic: a missed opportunity.

Overthinking and the result of restlessness and anxiety are also surprisingly common and, while it proves to be a great weakness in one's social and personal life, it becomes the source of lost opportunities and moments that one later regrets. But it could be easily overcome with a few routine exercises and a positive attitude.

Acceptance. The first step in overthinking and anxiousness is first and foremost to accept the issue. Only then could you go ahead to fix it. Nevertheless, while it is important to know that you are a remunerator, it is also vital that you understand that you are not alone and that there is no reason to fear. To think over is natural among many people today, and you could conquer it with a positive attitude.

The best time is the moment. Clearly, the best thing you can do without overthinking is stuck with the present. The mind can't think about stuff far away if it's going to be busy with the current. You also learn to appreciate the environment and currently fully enhance your success on any mission. And although it's much easier to say than to do, there are some strategies you can use every day to reduce the process of negative thinking.

Breathing is a good example. Learning how much this benefits would shock you. Just close your eyes and take a few minutes to breathe deeply. Watching closely and taking deep breaths helps you get in the moment and raises your head.

A good example is to meditate for consciousness. The basic idea is to remain silent and reflect on everything around you, and that has done wonderful things for many people. Close your eyes only once a day, and try to take in all of your surroundings. Listen to your feelings, but don't' interact,' and you may eventually try to reduce their' size.'

Therefore, slow down. Do all you do with your full awareness of it. Try and tell each action you take to push yourself to see the world. This will also motivate you to stay right now.

Be optimistic. When you feel comfortable with yourself and have self-esteem, you build up a positive outlook. You'd find yourself less inclined to overthink so that anything you do or say is better done. One of the first things you can do is get involved. Create a schedule for what to do for the day and continue to be successful. Doing things stop you from wandering away and, in fact, getting things done will lead to a huge increase in confidence through a feeling of accomplishment. You should also try to do something, at least once a day, you really are great. Whether you are an instrument player or you have outstanding video games talent, take a while off your schedule and do it. It's going to be a big help.

The change in life that you can make is to fake it. This may sound difficult, but it really works very well. Pretend you are a character you know, intelligence, cleverness, and self-assurance. You may know one of a TV show, a movie or a novel. Go ahead and deliver with certainty all you say, even if you're not sure of it or you're scared. When you make it faker, you will finally inherit the faith in real life.

Seeking to monitor all of your life's outcomes is, without a doubt, the main cause of remuneration because you are also forced to think feverishly about what to do at every stage in your life in fear of what might happen next. The best thing you can do is not to convince yourself. Realize that in your life, you have no say, and there's no reason to worry. The world has determined your fate, so you should make the most of every moment. Try to remember that before anything, you might hesitate to do it, and it will encourage you to stop and do it.

You can also make other timescales to take any decision. Whether it's to speak to someone or to make greater decisions in your life that may cause you to overthink, take a minute for the little ones, and a couple of days for the bigger ones in life. This would lead you to evaluate a decision rationally and to work to make the best possible option. Arm yourself when you make a decision and do it. It may be frightening, but at the end of the day, you find it satisfying.

CONCLUSION

We must always be aware of our thoughts and actions, but a person can influence himself negatively by overthrowing the object to which he may be obsessive or compelling, leading to self-destructive behaviour or delay. Very often, people are not sure how to solve these problems and can use jealousy and denial behaviours, which nourish their insecurities.

Often, how do we survive and rely on the power of self-belief? Can you honestly only believe in yourself and leave excessive thinking, worrying, and fear of failure behind? How can you learn to stop thinking to help you succeed? These are areas of concern both for the business world and for individuals and families, I hope this chapter will enable you to look at the inner light that wants you to believe in your ideas and approach to live honestly. Let us do this, for instance, by contemplating how self-belief is essential to make the right decisions, as a small business is perhaps faced with. You could be like most people and start enterprises to directly working on believing in yourself.

Excessive thought will kill any opportunity to take responsibility for the strength of self-belief.

People focus on worrying about every move in their job, probably overthinking the issues. Be more imaginative in your write down what surprising ways other people will find. With a simple plan and creative thought, the studies and presentations will improve.